CW00796754

Dietary Supplements
Pocket Companion

Dietary Supplements Pocket Companion

Pamela Mason
BSc, MSc, PhD, MRPharmS, RNutr
Pharmacist and Registered Nutritional
Writer and Consultant, Usk,
Monmouthshire, UK

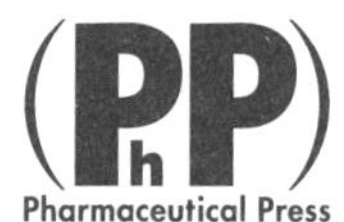

London • Chicago

Published by the Pharmaceutical Press
An imprint of RPS Publishing

1 Lambeth High Street, London SE1 7JN, UK
100 South Atkinson Road, Suite 200, Grayslake, IL 60030-7820, USA

(PhP) is a trade mark of RPS Publishing
RPS Publishing is the publishing organisation of the Royal Pharmaceutical Society of Great Britain

First published 2009

Typeset by Thomson Digital, Noida, India
Printed in Italy by Lego Print S.r.l.

ISBN 978 0 85369 761 9

A catalogue record for this book is available from the British Library

Contents

Preface vii
About the author xiii

Aloe vera 1
Alpha-lipoic acid 4
Antioxidants 7
Arginine 10
Bee pollen 13
Betaine 16
Biotin 18
Boron 21
Branched-chain amino acids 24
Brewers' yeast 26
Bromelain 28
Calcium 31
Carnitine 37
Carotenoids 40
Chitosan 42
Chlorella 44
Choline 46
Chondroitin 49
Chromium 51
Coenzyme Q10 54
Conjugated linoleic acid 57
Copper 60
Creatine 63
Dehydroepiandrosterone 67
Dong quai 70
Evening primrose oil 73
Fish oil 77
Flaxseed oil 82
Fluoride 84
Folic acid 86
Gamma-oryzanol 91
Garlic 93
Ginkgo biloba 96
Ginseng 99
Glucosamine 102
Grape seed extract 105
Green-lipped mussel 107
Green tea extract 109
Guarana 112
Hydroxycitric acid 115
5-Hydroxytryptophan 117
Iodine 121
Iron 124
Isoflavones 128
Kelp 131

Lecithin 133
Magnesium 135
Manganese 139
Melatonin 142
Methylsulfonylmethane 145
Molybdenum 147
Multivitamins 149
N-Acetylcysteine 153
Niacin 155
Nickel 159
Octacosanol 161
Pangamic acid 163
Pantothenic acid 165
Para-amino benzoic acid 168
Pycnogenol 170
Phosphatidylserine 172
Phytosterols 174
Potassium 176
Prebiotics 179
Probiotics 181
Psyllium 184
Pumpkin seeds 186
Quercetin 189
Resveratrol 193
Riboflavin 195
Royal jelly 198
S-Adenosyl methionine 201
Selenium 203
Shark cartilage 207
Silicon 209
Spirulina 211
Superoxide dismutase 213
Thiamine 215
Tin 219
Vanadium 221
Vitamin A 224
Vitamin B_6 228
Vitamin B_{12} 232
Vitamin C 236
Vitamin D 240
Vitamin E 244
Vitamin K 248
Zinc 251

Appendix 1: Guidance on safe upper levels of vitamins and minerals 255
Appendix 2: Drug and supplement interactions 257
Appendix 3: Additional resources 263

Index 267

Preface

What is Dietary Supplements Pocket Companion?

Dietary Supplements Pocket Companion is a quick reference, easily accessible text which is essentially a summary of the larger, fully referenced comprehensive text, *Dietary Supplements*. Like *Dietary Supplements, Dietary Supplements Pocket Companion* provides evidence-based, practice-relevant information but in a more concise and conveniently sized text, which a busy health professional can easily carry in a pocket or handbag.

As with the larger text, this publication attempts to evaluate the evidence for dietary supplements from published sources, including population-based observational studies, animal studies, controlled clinical trials, systematic reviews and meta-analyses. *Dietary Supplements Pocket Companion* summarises this evidence in tabular format with references to review literature for the reader who wishes to dig deeper. References to original clinical trials can be found in the fully referenced *Dietary Supplements* text.

Monographs

Dietary Supplements Pocket Companion contains 88 monographs on specific food supplement ingredients. The monographs follow the familiar format of the larger text. The information is based on the most recent quarterly update of *Dietary Supplements* at the time of going to press. These data are fully referenced and available at www.medicinescomplete.com. Only key references have been included in the Pocket Companion to keep the size to a minimum. Anyone interested in seeing the original source material can consult Medicines Complete, or the full reference work of *Dietary Supplements*.

The monographs are structured (where the supplement ingredient allows) as follows:

Description

States the type of substance; e.g. a vitamin, mineral, fatty acid, amino acid, enzyme, plant extract, etc.

Human requirements

Lists for different ages and sex (where established):

- UK Dietary Reference Values[1,2] and Safe Upper Levels. Dietary Reference Values (DRVs) includes the following:
  - EAR: Estimated Average Requirement. An assessment of the average requirement for energy or protein for a vitamin or mineral. About half the population will need more than the EAR, and half less.
  - LRNI: Lower Reference Nutrient Intake. The amount of protein, vitamin or mineral considered to be sufficient for the few people in a group who have low needs. Most people will need more than the LRNI and if people consistently consume less they may be at risk of deficiency of that nutrient.
  - RNI: Reference Nutrient Intake. The amount of protein, vitamin or mineral sufficient for almost every individual. This level of intake is much higher than many people need.
  - Safe Intake: A term used to indicate intake or range of intakes of a nutrient for which there is not enough information to estimate RNI, EAR or LRNI. It is considered to be adequate for almost everyone's needs but not large enough to cause undesirable effects.
  - Safe upper levels. These have been produced by the Food Standards Agency Expert Vitamin and Mineral Group[3] and defined as either the safe upper level or likely safe daily intake (where data are more limited) from supplements on a long term daily basis.

- Dietary Reference Values (DRVs) US Recommended Dietary Allowances (RDAs) and Tolerable Upper Intake Levels (ULs)
  - RDA: Recommended Dietary Allowance. The average amount of energy or a nutrient recommended to cover the needs of groups of healthy people.
  - Safe Intake and Adequate Daily Dietary Intakes. These are given for some vitamins and minerals where there is less information on which to base allowances, and figures are provided in the form of ranges.
  - Tolerable Upper Intake Levels. Defined by the Food and Nutrition Board of the US National Academy of Sciences[4–7] as the highest total level of a nutrient (diet plus supplements) which could be consumed safely on a daily basis, that is unlikely to cause adverse health effects to almost all individuals in the general population. As intakes rise above the TUL, the risk of adverse effects increases. The TUL describes long-term intakes, so an isolated dose above the TUL need not necessarily cause adverse effects. The TUL defines safety limits and is not a recommended intake for most people most of the time.

- World Health Organization (WHO) Reference Nutrient Intakes
- European Union Recommended Dietary Allowances (RDAs). This is an amount which is sufficient for most individuals. The EU RDA is used on dietary supplement labels.

Dietary intake

States amounts of nutrients provided by the average adult diet in the UK.[8]

Action

Describes the role of the substance in maintaining physiological function and identifies pharmacological actions where appropriate.

Dietary sources

Lists significant food sources.

Possible uses

Lists potential indications for use of each supplement (in table form) with the strength of the evidence.

Ideally the indication for a supplement should be based on a relationship that has been established by multiple randomised controlled trials of interventions on populations that are representative of the target of a recommendation, but this type of evidence may not always be available so the totality of the evidence should be considered.

The following criteria developed by the World Cancer Research Fund and modified by the World Health Organization (WHO)[9] are used to describe the strength of evidence in this report.

- *Convincing evidence*. Evidence based on epidemiological studies showing consistent associations between exposure and disease, with little or no evidence to the contrary. The available evidence is based on a substantial number of studies including prospective observational studies and where relevant, randomised controlled trials of sufficient size, duration and quality showing consistent effects. The association should be biologically plausible.
- *Probable evidence*. Evidence based on epidemiological studies showing fairly consistent associations between exposure and disease, but where there are perceived shortcomings in the available evidence or some evidence to the contrary, which precludes a more definite judgement. Shortcomings in the evidence may be any of the following: insufficient duration of trials (or studies); insufficient trials (or studies) available; inadequate sample sizes; incomplete follow-up. Laboratory evidence is usually supportive. Again, the association should be biologically plausible.
- *Possible evidence*. Evidence based mainly on findings from case-control and cross-sectional studies. Insufficient randomised controlled trials, observational studies or non-randomised controlled trials are available.

Evidence based on non-epidemiological studies, such as clinical and laboratory investigations, is supportive. More trials are required to support the tentative associations, which should also be biologically plausible.

- *Insufficient evidence*. Evidence based on findings of a few studies which are suggestive, but are insufficient to establish an association between exposure and disease. Limited or no evidence is available from randomised controlled trials. More well designed research is required to support the tentative associations.

Bioavailability

Provides data on bioavailability of the ingredient from a food supplement, where such data are available.

Precautions/contraindications

Lists diseases and conditions in which the substance should be avoided or used with caution.

Pregnancy and breastfeeding

Comments on safety or potential toxicity during pregnancy and lactation.

Adverse effects

Describes the risks that may accompany excessive intake, and signs and symptoms of toxicity.

Interactions

Lists drugs and other nutrients that may interact with the supplement. This includes drugs that affect vitamin and mineral status and supplements that influence drug metabolism.

Dose

Gives usual recommended dosage (if established).

References

References are mainly reviews and a few key clinical trials. The reader is referred to *Dietary Supplements* and Medicines Complete (www.medicinescomplete .com) for all original source material.

References

1. Department of Health. *Dietary Reference Values for Food Energy and Nutrients for the United Kingdom*. Report on Health and Social Subjects 41. Report of the Panel on Dietary Reference Values of the Committee on Medical Aspects of Food Policy; 1991.

2. Agarwal A, Allamaneni SS, Nallella KP, George AT, Mascha E. Correlation of reactive oxygen species levels with the fertilization rate after in vitro fertilization: a qualified meta-analysis. *Fertil Steril* 2005; 84: 228–231.

3. Expert Vitamin and Mineral Group. *Safe Upper Levels of Vitamins and Minerals*. 2003. Available from: http://www.food.gov.uk/multimedia/pdfs/vitmin2003.pdf. (accessed 6 February 2008).

4. Institute of Medicine Food and Nutrition Board. *Dietary reference intakes for calcium, phosphorus, magnesium, vitamin D and fluoride*. Washington DC: The National Academies Press; 1999.

5. Institute of Medicine Food and Nutrition Board. *Dietary reference intakes for thiamin, riboflavin, niacin, vitamin B_6, folate, vitamin B_{12}, pantothenic acid, biotin and choline*. Washington DC: The National Academies Press; 2000.

6. Institute of Medicine Food and Nutrition Board. *Dietary reference intakes for vitamin C, vitamin E, selenium and carotenoids*. Washington DC: The National Academies Press; 2000.

7. Institute of Medicine Food and Nutrition Board. *Dietary reference intakes for vitamin A, vitamin K, arsenic, boron, chromium, copper, iodine, iron, manganese, molybdenum, nickel, silicon, vanadium and zinc*. Washington DC: National Academies Press; 2002.

8. Henderson L, Irving K, Gregory J, Bates CJ, Prentice A, Parks J. *et al. National Diet and Nutrition Survey: adults aged 19 to 64 years. Volume 3. Vitamin and mineral intake and urinary analysis*. London: Stationery Office; 2003.

9. World Health Organization, Food and Agricultural Organization of the United Nations. *A model for establishing upper levels of intake for nutrients and related substances*. Report of a Joint FAO/WHO technical workshop on nutrient risk assessment, WHO Headquarters, Geneva, Switzerland, 2–6 May 2005; 2006.

About the author

Pamela Mason is a pharmaceutical and nutrition writer and consultant based in Usk, Monmouthshire. She qualified as a pharmacist at Manchester University and worked as a community pharmacist for several years before studying at King's College London, where she completed an MSc and PhD in nutrition. Her interest in food supplements began as a result of her studies in nutrition and her experience in community pharmacy where she was often asked questions about these products. She is the author of three other books, several open learning programmes and over 300 articles. She teaches nutrition to pharmacists at both undergraduate level and postgraduate level and gives conference presentations about supplements both in the UK and abroad.

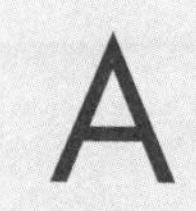

Aloe vera

Description

Aloe vera is the transparent gel from the pulp of the large blade-like leaves of the plant *Aloe vera*. Traditionally it has been used topically for thousands of years to treat skin infections, burns and wounds, and many other skin conditions. The dried latex from the inner lining of the leaf (aloes) has traditionally been used as an oral laxative.

Constituents

Aloe vera contains polysaccharides, tannins, sterols, saponins, vitamins, minerals, cholesterol, gamma-linolenic acid and arachidonic acid. Aloes contains anthraquinone compounds.

Action

- Topically, it acts as a moisturiser and reduces inflammation.
- Internally, it may act as an anti-inflammatory, hypoglycaemic and hyperlipidaemic agent.
- It also has anti-platelet activity.

Possible uses[1–3]

Health effect or disease risk	Strength of evidence
Aloe vera: topical	
Wound healing	PR
Psoriasis	P
Seborrhoeic dermatitis	P

continued

(*continued*)

Skin burns	P
Mouth ulcers	P
Infected wounds	I
Pressure ulcers	I
Aloe vera: oral	
Type 2 diabetes: ↓ blood glucose	P
↓ hyperlipidaemia	I
Irritable bowel syndrome	I
Ulcerative colitis	I
↑ absorption of vitamins C and E	P
Aloes (dried latex only): oral	
Laxative	C

C, convincing; I, insufficient; P, possible; PR, probable.

Precautions/contraindications

- *Aloe vera:* none established. Caution in diabetes mellitus because of potential hypoglycaemia.
- *Aloes:* not recommended. Contraindicated in abdominal disorders and ileus. Contraindicated in heart disease, kidney disease, electrolyte disturbance (or any condition where low potassium level is likely to cause problems).

Pregnancy/breastfeeding

- *Topical aloe vera:* is unlikely to be harmful.
- *Oral aloe vera:* not recommended because of theoretically causing uterine contractions.
- *Oral aloes:* contraindicated.

Adverse effects

- *Topical aloe vera:* allergy, skin redness, rash.
- *Oral aloe vera:* may lower blood sugar.
- *Oral aloes:* electrolyte disturbances, including hypokalaemia, failure of bowel function, dependency.

Interactions

Oral aloe vera: caution advised with drugs reducing blood sugar.

Dose

Aloe vera is available in the form of creams, gels, tablets, capsules and juice. The International Aloe Science Council (IASC) operates a voluntary approval scheme, which gives an official seal ('IASC certified') on products containing certified raw ingredients processed according to standard guidelines.

Used externally, aloe vera should be applied liberally as needed. The product should contain at least 20% aloe vera.

Used internally, there is no established dose. Product manufacturers suggest $^{1}/_{2}$ to $^{3}/_{4}$ cup of juice or one to two capsules three times a day. The juice in the product should ideally contain at least 98% aloe vera and no aloin. The safety of this regimen has not been proven.

References

1. Reynolds T. Aloe vera leaf gel: a review update. *J Ethnopharmacol* 1999; 68: 3–37.
2. Vogler BK, Ernst E. Aloe vera: a systematic review of its clinical effectiveness. *Br J Clin Pract* 1999; 49: 823–828.
3. Maenthaisong R, Chaiyakunapruk N, Niruntraporn S, Kongkaew C. The efficacy of aloe vera used for burn wound healing: a systematic review. *Burns* 2007; 33: 713–718.

Alpha-lipoic acid

Description

Alpha-lipoic acid (also known as alpha-lipoate, thioctic acid, lipoic acid, 2-dithiolane-3-pentatonic acid, 1,2-dithiolane-3-valeric acid) is a naturally occurring sulphur-containing cofactor. It is synthesised in humans.

Human requirements

It is not essential because the body synthesises it. However, some conditions (e.g. diabetes mellitus, liver cirrhosis and atherosclerosis) are associated with low levels of alpha-lipoic acid. It is difficult to obtain amounts used in clinical studies from foods.

Dietary sources

Kidney, heart, liver, spinach, broccoli, potatoes and brewers' yeast.

Action

- Antioxidant: alpha-lipoic acid is able to scavenge reactive oxygen species and other metabolites such as glutathione or vitamins. It is capable of thiol disulphide exchange.
- Cofactor for various enzymes (e.g. pyruvate dehydrogenase and 2-oxoglutarate dehydrogenase) in energy-producing metabolic reactions of the tricarboxylate or citrate cycle.
- Increases cellular uptake of glucose by recruiting the glucose transporter, GLUT4, to the cell membrane.
- May protect against mercury, arsenic and lead poisoning.

Possible uses[1–5]

Health effect or disease risk	Strength of evidence
Diabetes mellitus: Improves glucose metabolism	P P

Improves insulin sensitivity Diabetic neuropathy[a]	P P
Glaucoma	I
HIV	I
Dementia	I
Hypertension	I
Burning mouth syndrome	I
Age-related hearing loss (prevention)	I
Migraine (prevention)	I

I, insufficient; P, possible,
[a]High doses licensed in Germany for the treatment of diabetic neuropathy.

Bioavailability

Alpha-lipoic acid is 30% absorbed from supplements or foods and is reduced to dihydrolipoic acid in many tissues.

Precautions/contraindications

Diabetes mellitus and hypoglycaemia.

Pregnancy/breastfeeding

Insufficient data.

Adverse effects

No long-term safety studies. Skin rashes, gastrointestinal effects, nausea and headache reported. No serious side effects reported with doses up to 1800 mg daily.

Interactions

Theoretically:

- May increase risk of hypoglycaemia with insulin and hypoglycaemics.
- May decrease effectiveness of chemotherapy.
- May have additive effects with herbs causing hypoglycaemia (e.g. devil's claw, garlic, guar gum, ginseng, horse chestnut, psyllium).

Herbs with hyperglycaemic potential (e.g. ginger, gotu kola) may antagonise alpha-lipoic acid.

Dose

Not established. Studies use 600–1200 mg daily.

References

1. Kamenova P. Improvement of insulin sensitivity in patients with type 2 diabetes mellitus after oral administration of alpha-lipoic acid. *Hormones (Athens)* 2006; 5: 251–258.
2. Evans JL, Goldfine ID. Alpha-lipoic acid: a multifunctional antioxidant that improves insulin sensitivity in patients with type 2 diabetes. *Diabetes Technol Ther* 2000; 2: 401–413.
3. Wollin SD, Jones PJ. Alpha-lipoic acid and cardiovascular disease. *J Nutr* 2003; 133: 3327–3330.
4. Henriksen EJ. Exercise training and the antioxidant alpha-lipoic acid in the treatment of insulin resistance and type 2 diabetes. *Free Radic Biol Med* 2006; 40: 3–12.
5. Pershadsingh HA. Alpha-lipoic acid: physiologic mechanisms and indications for the treatment of metabolic syndrome. *Expert Opin Investig Drugs* 2007; 16: 291–302.

Antioxidants

Description

An antioxidant is a substance that delays or prevents oxidation.

Constituents

Nutrients with antioxidant properties include beta-carotene, vitamins A, C and E, and selenium, lycopene, lutein, zeaxanthin, flavonoids (e.g. anthocyanins, polyphenols, quercetin). The body also produces antioxidants, including alpha-lipoic acid, coenzyme Q10 and glutathione. In addition, copper and zinc are necessary to strengthen the body's own antioxidant protection system. Supplements marketed with antioxidant properties (in addition to the above) include carnitine, green tea, pine bark extract and resveratrol.

Dietary sources

Antioxidants are found principally in fruit, vegetables and other plant foods. The best sources tend to be the most colourful ones such as berries (e.g. blueberry, cranberry, raspberry, strawberry), kiwis and citrus fruit, legumes (e.g. broad beans, pinto beans, soya beans), walnuts, sunflower seeds, vegetables (e.g. kale, spinach, Brussels sprouts, beetroot, red cabbage, button mushrooms, peppers) and cereals (e.g. barley and oats).

Action

Antioxidants protect body tissues from the harmful effects of unstable oxygen molecules called free radicals. Free radicals are highly reactive substances that result from normal cellular oxidative metabolism and exposure to environmental insults, such as cigarette smoke, ultraviolet light, chemical pollutants and some medications. Left unchecked, these oxidant compounds can cause extensive cell damage to the body's cell membranes, proteins and DNA. Damage accumulates over time and can lead to a variety of health problems such as cardiovascular disease, cancer, macular degeneration, cataract, Parkinson's disease and Alzheimer's disease.

Possible uses

Observational studies suggest an inverse association between consumption of dietary antioxidants and risk of chronic disease such as Alzheimer's disease, arthritis, cancer, cardiovascular disease, cataracts, diabetes, macular degeneration and Parkinson's disease. In vitro studies have also shown that antioxidant compounds have a positive influence on various disease risk factors such as endothelial function, platelet aggregation, joint damage and cellular processes involved in carcinogenesis. However, placebo-controlled clinical trials have largely failed to show a benefit of antioxidant supplements and in some cases have suggested adverse effects.[1–4]

Health effect or disease risk	Strength of evidence (from RCTs)
Cardiovascular disease	I
Cancer	I
Cataract	P
Age-related macular degeneration	P
Arthritis	I
Mental performance	I
Physical performance	P
Pre-eclampsia	I
Asthma	I

I, insufficient; P, possible.
RCTs, randomised controlled trials.

Bioavailability

The bioavailability of vitamin C from supplements is approximately the same as that from foods. The bioavailability of vitamin E from supplements depends on the source: synthetic vitamin E (*d,l*-alpha-tocopherol) is absorbed less efficiently than natural vitamin E (*d*-alpha-tocopherol). The bioavailability of other antioxidants such as carotenoids and flavonoids is less clear.

Precautions/contraindications

There is no indication for supplements containing beta-carotene.

Pregnancy/breastfeeding

Insufficient data.

Adverse effects

A few studies have shown increased risk of cardiovascular disease and cancer with high dose antioxidant supplements. Beta-carotene supplementation (20 mg/day) has been associated with increased risk of cancer in smokers.

Interactions

One study found that antioxidants could block the favourable effects of statins (in combination with niacin).

Dose

Antioxidant vitamins and minerals are best avoided in doses exceeding the RDA (recommended daily allowance).

References

1. Vivekananthan DP, Penn MS, Sapp SK *et al.* Use of antioxidant vitamins for the prevention of cardiovascular disease: meta-analysis of randomized trials. *Lancet* 2003; 361: 2017–2023.

2. Agency for Healthcare Research and Quality. *Effect of supplemental antioxidants vitamin C, vitamin E and co-enzyme Q10 for the prevention and treatment of cardiovascular disease.* Evidence report/Technology Assessment: Number 83. AHRQ Publication Number 03-E042. Rockville, MD: AHRQ, 2003. Available from www.ahrq.gov/clinic/epcsums/antioxsum.htm (accessed 6 February 2008).

3. Agency for Healthcare Research and Quality. *Effect of the supplemental use of antioxidants vitamin C, vitamin E, and the coenzyme Q10 for the prevention and treatment of cancer.* Evidence report/Technology Assessment: Number 75. AHRQ Publication Number 04-E002. Rockville, MD: AHRQ, 2003. Available from www.ahrq.gov/clinic/epcsums/aoxcansum.htm (accessed 6 February 2008).

4. The Alpha Tocopherol B-CCPSG. The effect of vitamin E and beta carotene on the incidence of lung cancer in male smokers. *N Engl J Med* 1994; 330: 1029–1035.

Arginine

Description

This is a non-essential amino acid, which becomes essential during growth and catabolic states. Available as a supplement in the form of L-arginine.

Action

Involved in hepatic urea synthesis; substrate for nitric oxide (NO) synthase; precursor to NO (which causes vasodilatation in endothelial cells); antihypertensive and antioxidant; regulates extracellular pH; influences coagulation, fibrinolysis, blood viscosity, atherosclerosis and endothelial function.

Dietary sources

Meat, poultry, fish and dairy products.

Possible uses[1–4]

Health benefits	Evidence
Improved endothelial function and blood flow in cardiovascular disease	P
Improved walking and symptoms in peripheral arterial disease	P
Erectile dysfunction	I
Ergogenic acid in sports	I
Improved glucose metabolism	I
Improved immune function	I
Improved wound healing	P

I, insufficient; P, possible.

Bioavailability

No long-term data; dietary arginine is highly bioavailable.

Precautions/contraindications

Cardiovascular disease; herpes simplex; avoid in all medical conditions without medical supervision.

Pregnancy and breastfeeding

Avoid.

Adverse effects

Possibly sodium and water loss; possibly depletion of glycine and lysine levels; reports of gastrointestinal side effects.

Interactions

None reported. High doses may interfere with metabolism of other amino acids.

Dose

Not established. Doses used in studies: 3–20 g daily depending on condition (usually 3–6 g daily in cardiovascular disease).

References

1. Boger RH. L-Arginine therapy in cardiovascular pathologies: beneficial or dangerous? *Curr Opin Clin Nutr Metab Care* 2008; 11: 55–61.
2. Tousoulis D, Boger RH, Antoniades C, Siasos G, Stefanadi E, Stefanadis C. Mechanisms of disease: L-arginine in coronary atherosclerosis – a clinical perspective. *Nat Clin Pract Cardiovasc Med* 2007; 4: 274–283.
3. Boger RH. The pharmacodynamics of L-arginine. *J Nutr* 2007; 137(suppl 2): S1650–S1655.
4. McConell GK. Effects of L-arginine supplementation on exercise metabolism. *Curr Opin Clin Nutr Metab Care* 2007; 10: 46–51.

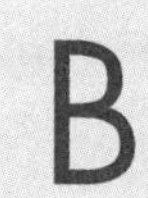

Bee pollen

Description

Bee pollen consists of flower pollen and nectar from male seed flowers.

Constituents

Bee pollen consists of protein, carbohydrates, minerals, essential fatty acids, B vitamins, vitamin C, flavonoids, and various amino acids, hormones, enzymes and coenzymes. The amounts of these substances present in various types of pollen are specific to the needs of the plant species; they are too small to be significant for humans.

Action

Bee pollen may have antioxidant and anti-inflammatory activity.

Possible uses[1–5]

Health effect or disease risk	Strength of evidence
Sports performance	I
Memory enhancement	I
Benign prostatic hyperplasia	I
Enhanced immune response	I
Hay fever/allergies	I

continued

(*continued*)

Premenstrual syndrome	I
Nosebleeds	I
Constipation and diarrhoea	I
Skin conditions (e.g. eczema, nappy rash) (topical)	I

I, insufficient.

Precautions/contraindications

Contraindicated in people with a known history of atopy or allergy to pollen or plant products because of the risk of hypersensitivity.

Pregnancy/breastfeeding

No problems reported but insufficient safety data.

Adverse effects

- Allergic reactions, including nausea, vomiting and anaphylaxis (may be fatal).
- May promote hyperglycaemia in diabetes.

Interactions

None documented.

Dose

Bee pollen is available in the form of capsules and powder.

The dose is not established. Product manufacturers tend to recommend doses of 500–1500 mg daily from capsules or half to one teaspoon of the powder.

References

1. Banskota AH, Tezuka Y, Kadota S. Recent progress in pharmacological research of propolis. *Phytother Res* 2001; 15: 561–571.
2. Burdock GA. Review of the biological properties and toxicity of bee propolis (propolis). *Food Chem Toxicol* 1998; 36: 347–363.
3. Khalil ML. Biological activity of bee propolis in health and disease. *Asian Pac J Cancer Prev* 2006; 7: 22–31.

4. Castaldo S, Capasso F. Propolis, an old remedy used in modern medicine. *Fitoterapia* 2002; 73(suppl 1): S1–S6.
5. Sforcin JM. Propolis and the immune system: a review. *J Ethnopharmacol* 2007; 113: 1–14.

Betaine

Description

Betaine is a cofactor in various methylation reactions and a major metabolite of choline.

Dietary sources

It is present in small amounts in cereals, seafood, wine and spinach.

Action

Betaine is a methyl group donor. It works with choline, vitamin B_{12} and also *S*-adenosyl methionine (SAM), a derivative of the amino acid methionine from which homocysteine is synthesised. It reduces homocysteine levels by remethylating homocysteine to produce methionine.

Betaine should not be confused with betaine hydrochloride, which is used as a source of hydrochloric acid, as a result of misleading claims that certain conditions are caused by insufficient gastric acid.

Possible uses[1–4]

Health effect or disease risk	Strength of evidence
Homocystinuria	PR
Dry mouth (topical)	P
Reduces plasma homocysteine	P
Reduces risk of cardiovascular disease	I

I, insufficient; P, possible; PR, probable.

Precautions/contraindications

Betaine should be avoided in patients with peptic ulcer.

Pregnancy/breastfeeding

No problems have been reported but there have not been sufficient studies to guarantee the safety of betaine in pregnant and breastfeeding women.

Adverse effects

Gastrointestinal irritation, including nausea and diarrhoea.

Interactions

None documented.

Dose

Betaine is available in the form of tablets and capsules.

Doses of 3 g twice a day have been used to lower homocysteine levels and in homocystinuria.

References

1. Craig SA. Betaine in human nutrition. *Am J Clin Nutr* 2004; 80: 539–549.
2. Olthof MR, Verhoef P. Effects of betaine intake on plasma homocysteine concentrations and consequences for health. *Curr Drug Metab* 2005; 6: 15–22.
3. Zeisel SH. Betaine supplementation and blood lipids: fact or artifact? *Nutr Rev* 2006; 64(2 Pt 1): 77–79.
4. Lawson-Yuen A, Levy HL. The use of betaine in the treatment of elevated homocysteine. *Mol Genet Metab* 2006; 88: 201–207.

Biotin

Description

Biotin is a sulphur-containing, water-soluble vitamin and a member of the vitamin B complex.

Human requirements

Dietary reference values (DRVs) for biotin					
Age	UK		USA		FAO/ WHO RNI (mcg/ day)
	Safe intake (mcg/day)	EVM (mcg/ day)	AI (mcg/ day)	TUL (mcg/ day)	
Males and females					
0–6 months			5	–	5
7–12 months			6	–	6
1–3 years			8	–	8
4–6 years			–	–	12
4–8 years			12	–	–
7–9 years			–	–	20
9–13 years			20	–	–
10–18 years			–	–	25
14–18 years			25	–	–
19–50 years			30	–	45

51+ years			30	–	45
11–50+ years	10–20	970	–	–	–
Pregnancy			30	–	30
Lactation			35	–	35

EU RDA = 150 mcg.
AI, adequate intake; EU RDA, European Union recommended daily allowance; EVM, likely safe daily intake from supplements alone; RNI, reference nutrient intake; TUL, tolerable upper intake level (not determined for biotin).

Dietary sources

The best sources of biotin are liver, kidney, eggs, soya beans and peanuts. Meat, wholegrain cereals, wholemeal bread, milk and cheese are also good sources. Green vegetables contain very little biotin.

Action

Biotin is an integral part of enzymes involved in bicarbonate-dependent carboxylation reactions. Biotin enzymes are involved in gluconeogenesis, fatty acid synthesis, propionate metabolism and catabolism of amino acids.

Possible uses[1,2]

Health effect or disease risk	Strength of evidence
Prevention and treatment of biotin deficiency	C
Biotinidase deficiency	C
Brittle nails	I
Acne	I
Candida infection	I
Reduced blood glucose and insulin in diabetes	I
Peripheral neuropathy	I
Alopecia areata	I

C, convincing; I, insufficient.

Bioavailability

Oral biotin seems to be 100% absorbed.[3]

Precautions/contraindications

No problems have been reported.

Pregnancy/breastfeeding

No problems have been reported.

Adverse effects

None reported.

Interactions

Drugs

Anticonvulsants (carbamazepine, phenobarbital, phenytoin and primidone): requirements for biotin may be increased.

Dose

Biotin is available in the form of tablets and capsules. However, it is available mainly in multi-vitamin preparations.

The dose is not established. Dietary supplements provide 100–300 mcg daily.

References

1. Expert Group on Vitamins and Minerals. Biotin. In: *Safe Upper Levels of Vitamins and Minerals*, 2003; 36–41. London: Food Standards Agency. Available at: www.food.gov.uk/multimedia/pdfs/vitmin2003.pdf (accessed 6 February 2008).
2. Fernandez-Mejia C. Pharmacological effects of biotin. *J Nutr Biochem* 2005; 16: 424–427.
3. Zempleni J, Mock DM. Bioavailability of biotin given orally to humans in pharmacologic doses. *Am J Clin Nutr* 1999; 69: 504–508.

Boron

Description

Boron is an ultratrace mineral.

Human requirements

Boron is essential in plants and some animals and evidence of essentiality is accumulating in humans, although requirements have not so far been defined.

Dietary sources

- Foods of plant origin, especially non-citrus fruit, leafy vegetables and nuts, are rich sources.
- Beer, wine and cider contain significant amounts.
- Meat, fish and poultry contain small amounts.

Action

- Important in calcium metabolism.
- Can affect the composition, structure and strength of bone.
- May influence the metabolism of calcium, copper, magnesium, phosphorus, potassium and vitamin D.
- Affects the activity of certain enzymes.
- Affects brain function; boron deprivation appears to depress mental alertness.

Possible uses[1–4]

Health effect or disease risk	Strength of evidence
Prevents calcium loss	P
Prevents bone demineralisation	P

continued

(continued)

Elevates oestrogen levels	P
Improves cognitive function	P
Osteoarthritis	I
Short-term memory	I
Attention span	I
Hand–eye coordination	I

I, insufficient; P, possible.

Bioavailability

One study showed that supplemental boron (3 mg daily) increased plasma boron concentration by one and a half times.[5]

Precautions/contraindications

None known.

Pregnancy/breastfeeding

Limited safety data during pregnancy and breastfeeding.

Adverse effects

Non-toxic when administered orally at doses contained in food supplements.

High oral doses (> 100 mg daily) are associated with disturbances in appetite and digestion, nausea, vomiting, diarrhoea, dermatitis and lethargy.

Interactions

Riboflavin: large doses of boron may increase excretion of riboflavin.
Magnesium: boron supplementation may reduce urinary magnesium excretion and increase serum magnesium concentrations.

Dose

Not established.
Dietary supplements provide, on average, 3 mg per daily dose.

References

1. Expert Group on Vitamins and Minerals. *Safe Upper Levels of Vitamins and Minerals*. London: Food Standards Agency, 2003. Available at: www.food.gov.uk (accessed 13 April 2008).

2. Newnham RE. Essentiality of boron for healthy bones and joints. *Environ Health Perspect* 1994; 102(suppl 7): 83–85.

3. Nielsen FH. The justification for providing dietary guidance for the nutritional intake of boron. *Biol Trace Elem Res* 1998; 66: 319–330.

4. Nielsen FH. Biochemical and physiologic consequences of boron deprivation in humans. *Environ Health Perspect* 1994; 102(suppl 7): 59–63.

5. Hunt CD, Herbel JL, Nielsen FH. Metabolic responses of postmenopausal women to supplemental dietary boron and aluminum during usual and low magnesium intake: boron, calcium, and magnesium absorption and retention and blood mineral concentrations. *Am J Clin Nutr* 1997; 65: 803–813.

Branched-chain amino acids

Description

Branched-chain amino acids (BCAAs) (i.e. L-leucine, L-isoleucine, L-valine) are a group of essential amino acids. They are found in muscle and account for a third of all amino acids in muscle protein.

Action

Precursors for synthesis of proteins; serve as an energy source (if necessary); used directly by skeletal muscle (no requirement for prior gluconeogenesis in the liver); may compete with serotonin transport in brain, so improving mental and physical performance.

Possible uses[1,2]

Health benefits	Evidence
Improve physical performance during exercise	I
Enhance muscle strength in amyotrophic lateral sclerosis	I
Anorexia/cachexia	I

I, insufficient.

Precautions/contraindications

Avoid in hepatic/renal impairment (except under rigorous medical supervision in a medical setting).

Pregnancy/breastfeeding

Inadequate data to guarantee safety.

Adverse effects

No long-term safety data. Large doses of BCAAs (> 20 g) may increase plasma ammonia and impair water absorption, causing gastrointestinal discomfort.

Interactions

None reported. BCAAs may compete with aromatic amino acids (e.g. phenylalanine, tyrosine, tryptophan) for transport into the brain.

Dose

Not established. Supplements (tablets, powders) provide 7–20 g per dose.

References

1. Gleeson M. Interrelationship between physical activity and branched-chain amino acids. *J Nutr* 2005; 135(suppl): S1591–S1595.
2. Bianchi G, Marzocchi R, Agostini F, Marchesini G. Update on nutritional supplementation with branched-chain amino acids. *Curr Opin Clin Nutr Metab Care* 2005; 8: 83–87.

Brewers' yeast

Description

Brewers' yeast is *Saccharomyces cerevisiae.*

Constituents

It is a good source of B vitamins (particularly folic acid), iron, chromium (known as glucose tolerance factor – GTF), zinc and copper.

Possible uses

Health effect or disease risk	Strength of evidence
Source of B vitamins	C
Source of chromium	C
Controls blood glucose levels	P
Hypercholesterolaemia	P
Diarrhoea due to *Clostridium difficile*[1]	P
Acne	I
Exercise performance	I
Athletic recovery/free radical stress	I

C, convincing; I, insufficient; P, possible.

Bioavailability

No data.

Precautions/contraindications

- Patients taking monoamine oxidase inhibitors (MAOIs).
- Gout (because of high purine content).

Pregnancy/breastfeeding

No problems reported.

Adverse effects

None reported except occasional flatulence.

Interactions

MAOIs: may provoke hypertensive crisis.

Dose

Brewers' yeast is available in the form of tablets and powder.

The dose is not established. In clinical studies for blood sugar control, 5–30 g of GTF-containing brewers' yeast was taken daily.

Reference

1. Sargent G, Wickens H. Brewers' yeast in *C. difficile* infection: probiotic or B group vitamins. *Pharmacy J* 2004; 273: 230–231.

Bromelain

Description

Bromelain is the name for the protease enzymes extracted from the family Bromeliaceae, usually from the pineapple, which is one member of Bromeliaceae.

Constituents

Bromelains are sulphydryl proteolytic enzymes, including several proteases. In addition, bromelain also contains small amounts of non-proteolytic enzymes (including acid phosphatase, peroxidase and cellulase), polypeptide protease inhibitors and organically bound calcium.

Dietary sources

Although pineapple is a good source of bromelain, the bromelain is concentrated mainly in the stem, which is less tasty than the fruit, so eating pineapple does not provide much bromelain.

Action

Bromelain is an anti-inflammatory agent and thought to act through antagonism of proinflammatory mediators. It inhibits the enzyme thromboxane synthase, which converts prostaglandin H_2 into proinflammatory prostaglandins and thromboxanes. Bromelain also stimulates the breakdown of fibrin, which stimulates proinflammatory prostaglandins responsible for fluid retention and clot formation. It also appears to promote the conversion of plasminogen to plasmin, causing an increase in fibrinolysis.

Possible uses[1]

Health effect or disease risk	Strength of evidence
Sinusitis	I
Enhances action of antibiotics	I
Musculoskeletal injuries	P
Arthritis	P
Bruising and swelling	P
Diarrhoea	I
Chronic venous insufficiency	I
Ulcerative colitis	I
Haemorrhoids	I
Menstrual pain	P

I, insufficient; P, possible.

Bioavailability

The research on the bioavailability of bromelain is limited. However, absorption has been demonstrated in both rats[2] and humans[3] as evidenced by the appearance of bromelain in serum.

Precautions/contraindications

- Caution with anticoagulants and anti-platelet agents.
- Contraindicated in pineapple allergy.

Pregnancy/breastfeeding

No data.

Adverse effects

Rare reports of nausea, vomiting, diarrhoea and menorrhagia. May inhibit platelet aggregation.

Interactions

- Bromelain may increase absorption and levels of amoxicillin and tetracyclines.
- Theoretically, there is increased bleeding risk with anticoagulants.

Dose

Bromelain is available in the form of tablets, capsules and powders. A variety of designations has been used to indicate the activity of bromelain. These include rorer units (ru), gelatine-dissolving units (gdu) and milk-clotting units (mcu). One gram of bromelain standardised to 2000 mcu would be approximately equal to 1 g with 1200 gdu of activity or 8 g with 100 000 ru activity.[1]

The dose is not established. Dietary supplements provide 125–500 mg in a dose.

References

1. Maurer HR. Bromelain: biochemistry, pharmacology and medical use. *Cell Mol Life Sci* 2001; 58: 1234–1245.
2. White RR, Crawley FE, Vellini M, Rovati LA. Bioavailability of ^{125}I bromelain after oral administration to rats. *Biopharm Drug Dispos* 1988; 9: 397–403.
3. Castell JV, Friedrich G, Kuhn CS, Poppe GE. Intestinal absorption of undegraded proteins in men: presence of bromelain in plasma after oral intake. *Am J Physiol* 1997; 273(1 Pt 1): G139–G146.

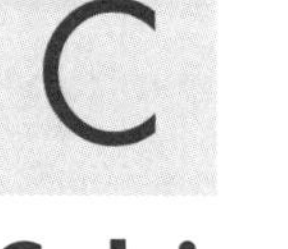

Calcium

Description

Calcium is an essential mineral.

Human requirements

DRVs for calcium							
Age	UK				US		WHO
	LNRI (mg/day)	EAR (mg/day)	RNI (mg/day)	EVM (mg/day)	AI (mg/day)	TUL (mg/day)	RNI (mg/day)
0–6 months	240	400	525		210	–	300[a]
7–12 months	240	400	525		270	–	400
1–3 years	200	275	350		500	2500	500
4–6 years	275	350	450		–	–	600
4–8 years	–	–	–		800	2500	–
7–10 years	325	425	550		800	–	700[b]
9–18 years	–	–	–		1300	2500	–

continued

(continued)

Males							
11–14 years	450	750	1000		–	–	1300[c]
15–18 years	450	750	1000		–	–	1300
19–24 years	400	525	700	1500	–	2500	1000
25–50 years	400	525	700	1500	1000	2500	1000
50+ years	400	525	700	1500	1200	2500	1000[f]
Females							
11–14 years	480	625	800		–	–	1300[c]
15–18 years	480	625	800		–	–	1300
19–50 years	400	525	700	1500	1000	2500	1000
50+ years	400	525	700	1500	1200	2500	1300
Pregnancy	[a]	[a]	[a]		1000[d]	2500	1200[g]
Lactation			+550		1000[d]	2500	1000

EU RDA = 800 mg.
AI, adequate intake.
[a]No increment
[b]7–9 years.
[c]10–14 years.
[d]≤ 18 years, 1300 mg
[e]400 mg for cows' milk fed.
[f]1300 mg for men > 65 years
[g]Third trimester.
AI, adequate intake; EAR, estimated average requirement; EU RDA, European Union recommended daily allowance; EVM, likely safe daily intake from supplements alone; LNRI, lower reference nutrient intake; RNI, reference nutrient intake; TUL, tolerable upper intake level.
Note: the National Osteoporosis Society has produced separate guidelines for recommended daily calcium intake as follows: 7–12 years, 800 mg; 13–19 years, 1000 mg; men 20–45 years, 1000 mg; men >45 years, 1500 mg; women 20–45 years, 1000 mg; women >45 years, 1500 mg; women >45 years (using hormone replacement therapy), 1000 mg; pregnant and breastfeeding women, 1200 mg; pregnant and breastfeeding teenagers, 1500 mg.

Dietary sources

Milk, cheese and other milk products (except butter and cream), some leafy green vegetables (e.g. broccoli, kale, spinach), fish eaten with their soft bones (e.g. sardines, canned salmon, pilchards, anchovies), soya beans (including tofu, soya milk), legumes (e.g. lentils, kidney beans, chickpeas), and calcium fortified products (e.g. calcium-fortified orange juice and bread).

Action

Calcium is a major mineral, which makes up 1.5–2% of the body weight. Of this amount, 99% is present in bones and teeth; the remaining 1% is found in soft tissues and body fluids, and serves a number of functions not related to bone structure. Calcium is important in blood coagulation, transmission of nerve impulses, contraction of muscle fibres, myocardial function and activation of enzymes.

Possible uses[1]

Health effect or disease risk	Strength of evidence
Improving bone mineral density: During the first three decades of life where dietary calcium intake is low In youngsters with adequate calcium intakes In premenopausal women	 C P P
Reducing bone loss: In early postmenopausal women In later postmenopausal women	 I P
Reduced risk of fracture in older people	C (with vitamin D)
Corticosteroid-induced osteoporosis	C (with vitamin D)
Hypertension	C (small but significant effect on systolic blood pressure)
Cancer Reduced risk of colon cancer Increased risk of prostate cancer	 P P
Reduced menstrual pain	PR
Pre-eclampsia	P
Weight management	
Reduced weight gain in middle age	P
Loss of body weight	I

C, convincing; I, insufficient; P, possible; PR, probable.

Bioavailability

Calcium carbonate is the most cost-effective form of calcium supplement.

Calcium citrate is equally well absorbed (a few studies have shown it to be better absorbed than calcium carbonate) and is the supplement of choice for individuals with achlorhydria or who are taking histamine H_2-receptor antagonists or protein pump inhibitors.

Calcium lactate and calcium gluconate are less concentrated forms of calcium and are not practical oral supplements.

Calcium absorption can be reduced by oxalates (e.g. in spinach) or phytates (e.g. in wheat bran). High protein and/or high sodium diets increase urinary calcium excretion.

Precautions/contraindications

Avoid in hypercalcaemia, hypercalcuria and renal impairment.

Pregnancy/breastfeeding

No problems reported.

Adverse effects

In high doses (above the tolerable upper intake level or TUL) calcium can cause constipation, hypercalcaemia and urinary stone formation.

Interactions

Drugs

Alcohol: excessive alcohol intake may reduce calcium absorption.
Aluminium-containing antacids: may reduce calcium absorption.
Anticonvulsants: may reduce serum calcium levels.
Bisphosphonates: calcium may reduce absorption of etidronate; give 2 hours apart.
Cardiac glycosides: concurrent use with parenteral calcium preparations may increase risk of cardiac arrhythmias (ECG monitoring recommended).
Corticosteroids: may reduce serum calcium levels.
Laxatives: prolonged use of laxatives may reduce calcium absorption.
Loop diuretics: increased excretion of calcium.
4-Quinolones: may reduce absorption of 4-quinolones; give 2 hours apart.
Tamoxifen: calcium supplements may increase the risk of hypercalcaemia (a rare side effect of tamoxifen therapy); calcium supplements are best avoided.
Tetracyclines: may reduce absorption of tetracyclines; give 2 hours apart.
Thiazide diuretics: may reduce calcium excretion.

Nutrients

Fluoride: may reduce absorption of fluoride and vice versa; give 2 hours apart.
Iron: calcium carbonate or calcium phosphate may reduce absorption of iron; give 2 hours apart (absorption of iron in multiple formulations containing iron and calcium is not significantly altered).
Vitamin D: increased absorption of calcium and increased risk of hypercalcaemia; may be advantageous in some individuals.
Zinc: may reduce absorption of zinc.

Dose

- The dose for potential prevention of osteoporosis is 1000–1200 mg (as elemental calcium) daily with 800 units of cholecalciferol. The maximum dose of elemental calcium that should be taken at a time is 500 mg.
- Calcium carbonate should be taken with a meal to ensure optimal absorption.
- Calcium citrate can be taken without food.
- Supplementation may be required in the following:
  - Those aged 65 years and over who are confined to their own homes or care homes.
  - Postmenopausal women younger than 65 years in whom lifestyle modification is unsustainable.
  - Secondary prevention of osteoporotic fractures in postmenopausal women (this is covered by the 2005 NICE guidelines[2]).
  - Prevention of osteoporotic fractures in patients taking glucocorticoids.

Calcium content of commonly used calcium salts

Calcium salt	Calcium (mg/g)	Calcium (%)
Calcium amino acid chelate	180	18
Calcium carbonate	400	40
Calcium chloride	272	27.2
Calcium glubionate	65	6.5
Calcium gluconate	90	9
Calcium lactate	130	13
Calcium lactate gluconate	129	13
Calcium orotate	210	21
Calcium phosphate (dibasic)	230	23

Note: calcium lactate and gluconate are more efficiently absorbed than calcium carbonate (particularly in patients with achlorhydria).

References

1. Straub DA. Calcium supplementation in clinical practice: a review of forms, doses, and indications. *Nutr Clin Pract* 2007; 22: 286–296.

2. National Institute for Health and Clinical Excellence. *Osteoporosis – Secondary Prevention. The clinical effectiveness and cost effectiveness of technologies for the secondary prevention of osteoporotic fractures in postmenopausal women.* London: NICE, 2005.

Carnitine

Description

Carnitine is the generic term for a number of compounds including L-carnitine (natural form), D-carnitine (synthetic form), DL-carnitine, acetyl-L-carnitine and propionyl-L-carnitine. It is synthesised by the liver and kidneys from the amino acids, lysine and methionine. L-Carnitine is the active form in the body.

Constituents

Dietary supplements contain L-carnitine or a DL-carnitine mixture.

Human requirements

There is no proof of a dietary need. Carnitine is synthesised in sufficient quantities to meet human requirements.

Dietary sources

Animal foods: meat (principally red meat), fish, poultry and milk (predominantly in the whey fraction). L-Carnitine is the form found in food. Mixed omnivorous diets provide 60–180 mg carnitine daily. Vegetarian diets provide 10–12 mg.

Action

- Plays a critical role in energy production.
- Regulates transport of long-chain fatty acids across cell membranes to the mitochondria.
- Facilitates beta-oxidation of long-chain fatty acids and ketoacids.
- Transports acyl-CoA compounds.

Possible uses[1]

Health effect or disease risk	Strength of evidence
CVD: Improves symptoms of angina Improves cardiovascular outcomes post-MI Improves outcomes in CHF Improves outcomes in PVD Improves lipid profile	 P P P P P
Athletic performance	I
Chronic fatigue syndrome	I
Reduces deterioration in Alzheimer's disease	I
Ameliorates fatigue in cancer	P
Improves symptoms of diabetic neuropathy	P
Slows progression of HIV	I
Improves male infertility	I

I, insufficient; P, possible.
CHF, congestive heart failure; CVD, cardiovascular disease; MI, myocardial infarction; PVD, peripheral vascular disease.

Bioavailability

Bioavailability of an oral dose is 5–20% (about 16% at 2 g oral dose; about 5% at 6 g oral dose).[2] Supplemental carnitine raises plasma carnitine but also increases renal clearance. Muscle carnitine is increased with long-term supplementation, but after supplementation of not less than 2 weeks' duration.

Precautions/contraindications

Avoid use of D-carnitine

Pregnancy/breastfeeding

No problems reported; insufficient data.

Adverse effects

Nausea, vomiting, diarrhoea (at doses >3 g/day)

Interactions

Drugs

Anticonvulsants: increased excretion of carnitine.
Carboplatin: increased excretion of carnitine
Pivampicillin: increased excretion of carnitine.
Pivmecillinam: increased excretion of carnitine.

Dose

Dose not established. Studies have used 1–6 g/day. Supplements contain L-carnitine, acetyl-L-carnitine and propionyl-L-carnitine. Evidence of safety is good at intakes of up to 2 g/day.[3]

References

1. Evangeliou A, Vlassopoulos D. Carnitine metabolism and deficit – when supplementation is necessary? *Curr Pharm Biotechnol* 2003; 4: 211–219.
2. Bain MA, Milne RW, Evans AM. Disposition and metabolite kinetics of oral L-carnitine in humans. *J Clin Pharmacol* 2006; 46: 1163–1170.
3. Hathcock JN, Shao A. Risk assessment for carnitine. *Regul Toxicol Pharmacol* 2006; 46: 23–28.

Carotenoids

Description

Carotenoids are natural pigments found in plants, including fruit and vegetables, giving them their bright colour.

Constituents

About 600 carotenoids have been identified. Significant carotenoids in human nutrition are alpha-carotene, astaxanthin, beta-carotene, cryptoxanthin, lycopene, lutein and zeaxanthin.

Dietary sources

Alpha-carotene: palm oil, maize, carrots and pumpkin.
Beta-carotene: apricots, carrots, kale, mango, spinach.
Lycopene: red fruit, such as tomatoes (particularly cooked and pureed tomatoes), guava, watermelon, apricots, peaches and red grapefruit.
Lutein and zeaxanthin: dark-green vegetables, red pepper and pumpkin.
Cryptoxanthin: mangoes, oranges and peaches.

Action

Carotenoids act principally as antioxidants and on immune function. Some carotenoids (e.g. alpha-carotene, beta-carotene, cryptoxanthin) act as precursors for vitamin A.

Possible uses (supplements)[1]

Health effect or disease risk	Strength of evidence (from RCTs)
Cancer:	
Colon	I
Breast	I
Cervix	I
Lung	I
Prostate (lycopene)	P

Cardiovascular disease	I
Cataract (lutein/zeaxanthin)	P

I, insufficient; P, possible.
RCTs, randomised controlled trials.

Bioavailability

Beta-carotene: the efficiency of absorption is usually 20–50%, but can be as low as 10% when intake is high. The conversion of beta-carotene to retinol is regulated by the individual's vitamin A stores and the amount ingested; conversion efficiency varies from 2:1 at low intakes to 12:1 at higher intakes. On average, 25% of absorbed beta-carotene appears to remain intact and 75% is converted to retinol.

Precautions/contraindications

No problems have been reported.

Pregnancy/breastfeeding

No problems reported.

Adverse effects

Generally non-toxic. Intake of >30 mg daily (either from commercial supplements or from tomato or carrot juice) may lead to hypercarotenaemia, which is characterised by a yellowish coloration of the skin (including the palms of the hands and soles of the feet), and a very high concentration of carotenoids in the plasma. This is harmless and reversible and gradually disappears when excessive intake of carotenoids is corrected.

Interactions

None reported.

Dose

Beta-carotene, lutein, lycopene and mixed carotenoids are available in the form of tablets and capsules. Beta-carotene should not be recommended as a single supplement.

Reference

1. Rao AV, Rao LG. Carotenoids and human health. *Pharmacol Res* 2007; 55: 207–216.

Chitosan

Description

Chitosan is an amino polysaccharide with a chemical structure similar to cellulose.

It is extracted from chitin, a structural component of crustacean shells, shrimps, prawns and lobsters, the exoskeleton of insects and the cell walls of fungi. Chitin is deacetylated to produce chitosan.

Action

Binds fat molecules as a result of its ionic nature and may prevent fat absorption.

Possible uses[1,2]

Health effect or disease risk	Strength of evidence
Prevents fat absorption	P
Promotes weight loss	I
Lowers total cholesterol	I
Lowers blood glucose	I

I, insufficient; P, possible.

Bioavailability

Chitosan cannot be hydrolysed by human digestive enzymes. In the acidic environment of the upper gastrointestinal tract, chitosan is solubilised and has a positive charge, so binds with negatively charged molecules such as fat and bile.

Precautions/contraindications

- Avoid in individuals with gastrointestinal malabsorption.
- Avoid in individuals with allergy to shellfish.

Pregnancy/breastfeeding

No problems reported. Weight loss should not be attempted during pregnancy.

Adverse effects

May reduce absorption of fat-soluble vitamins and minerals; possible negative consequences of long-term administration on bone health and nutritional deficiencies; may negatively influence intestinal flora, thus affecting bile and lipid metabolism, and promoting growth of intestinal pathogens.

Interactions

None reported, but as a type of fibre, chitosan could reduce absorption of medicines.

Dose

Not established. Manufacturers recommend taking up to 1500 mg daily with food, particularly fatty food. Take with plenty of fluid.

References

1. Mhurchu CN, Dunshea-Mooij C, Bennett D, Rodgers A. Effect of chitosan on weight loss in overweight and obese individuals: a systematic review of randomized controlled trials. *Obes Rev* 2005; 6: 3–4.
2. Liao F-H, Shieh M-J, Chang N-C, Chien Y-W. Chitosan supplementation lowers serum lipids and maintains normal calcium, magnesium and iron status in hyperlipidemic patients. *Nutr Res* 2007; 27: 146–151.

Chlorella

Description

Chlorella species is a single-cell freshwater alga.

Constituents

Rich in chlorophyll; claimed to be a valuable source of amino acids, nucleic acids, vitamins and minerals, but content varies with growing environment, harvesting and growing.

Action

Claimed to have antiviral and anti-cancer activity and to boost the immune system.

Possible uses[1]

Health effect or disease risk	Strength of evidence
Tonic	P
Source of nutrients: carotenoids, riboflavin, vitamin B_{12}, iron and zinc	PR
Relieves symptoms of fibromyalgia	P
Improves tolerance to chemotherapy	I
Wound healing	I
Improved digestive and bowel function	I
Slows ageing	I
Reduces high blood pressure	I
Growth and repair of tissues	I

Improves condition of hair, nails and skin	I
Boosts immune function	I
Removes toxins	I

I, insufficient; P, possible; PR, probable.

Bioavailability

No data.

Precautions/contraindications

No problems reported.

Pregnancy/breastfeeding

No problems reported.

Adverse effects

None reported.

Interactions

None reported.

Dose

- *Chlorella* is available in the form of tablets, capsules, liquid extracts and powder.
- The dose is not established. Dietary supplements provide 500–3000 mg of the intact organism per daily dose.

Reference

1. Merchant RE, Andre CA. A review of recent clinical trials of the nutritional supplement *Chlorella pyrenoidosa* in the treatment of fibromyalgia, hypertension, and ulcerative colitis. *Altern Ther Health Med* 2001; 7: 79–91.

Choline

Description

Choline is a quaternary amine widely distributed in foods. It can be synthesised endogenously from phosphatidylethanolamine. Most choline in the body is found in phospholipids such as phosphatidylcholine (lecithin) and sphingomyelin.

Human requirements

It is essential for several animals, but not established as essential for humans. The US daily recommended intake (DRI) is 550 mg/day for men and 425 mg/day for women, with lower amounts for children, together with an upper intake level of 3.5 g daily for adults aged over 18 years.

Dietary intake

Estimated dietary intake in the UK is 250–500 mg daily.

Dietary sources

Choline is widely distributed in foods (mainly in the form of lecithin). The richest sources of choline are brewers' yeast, egg yolk, liver, wheatgerm, soya beans, kidney and brain. Oats, peanuts, beans and cauliflower contain significant amounts.

Action

- Source of labile methyl groups for transmethylation reactions.
- A component of other molecules (e.g. acetylcholine, phosphatidylcholine [lecithin] and sphingomyelin).
- Structural constituents of cell membranes and plasma lipoproteins, platelet-activating factor and plasmalogen (a phospholipid found in highest concentrations in cardiac muscle membranes).
- Needed for normal neural tube closure in mammals.

- Critical for brain development in animals.
- Important for cell growth, regulation and function.

Possible uses[1,2]

Health effect or disease risk	Strength of evidence
Increases acetylcholine concentration in the brain	I
Prevents deterioration in Alzheimer's disease and dementia	I
Improves memory	I
Improves athletic performance	I
Reduces plasma homocysteine	P
Reduces lipid peroxidation	P
Prevents CVD	I

I, insufficient; P, possible.
CVD, cardiovascular disease.

Bioavailability

No data for supplements.

Precautions/contraindications

No problems reported.

Pregnancy/breastfeeding

No problems reported.

Adverse effects

With doses >10 g/day, diarrhoea, nausea, dizziness, sweating, salivation, depression and increased P–R interval on ECGs.

Interactions

None established.

Dose

Not established. Dietary supplements generally provide 250–500 mg per dose (choline chloride provides 80% choline and choline tartrate 50% choline).

References

1. Zeisel SH. Nutritional importance of choline for brain development. *J Am Coll Nutr* 2004; 23(suppl): S621–S626.
2. Zeisel SH. Choline: an essential nutrient for humans. *Nutrition* 2000; 16: 669–671.

Chondroitin

Description

Chondroitin is the principal glycosaminoglycan found in cartilage. It is synthesised endogenously and secreted by chondrocytes. Supplements are derived from bovine trachea or shark cartilage.

Constituents

High-molecular-weight glycosaminoglycans and disaccharide polymers composed of equimolar amounts of D-glucuronic acid, D-acetylgalactosamine and sulphates in 10–30 disaccharide units. (Glycosaminoglycans are the substances in which collagen fibres are embedded in cartilage.)

Action

- Absorbs water, adding to the thickness and elasticity of cartilage and its ability to absorb and distribute compressive forces.
- Controls formation of new cartilage matrix, by stimulating chondrocyte metabolism and synthesis of collagen and proteoglycan.
- Inhibits degradative enzymes (elastase and hyaluronidase), which break down cartilage matrix and synovial fluid, contributing to cartilage destruction and loss of joint function.

Possible uses[1,2]

Health effect or disease risk	Strength of evidence
Relieves osteoarthritis	PR
Protects joints and tendons from sports injuries	P
Secondary prevention of coronary events in patients with a history of CHD	I

I, insufficient; P, possible; PR, probable.
CHD, coronary heart disease.

Bioavailability

Appears to be effectively absorbed in the intestine.[3] Absorption depends on chain length.

Precautions/contraindications

No problems reported. Allergy to cartilaginous material.

Pregnancy/breastfeeding

Effects unknown.

Adverse effects

No known serious side effects. Rare reports of headaches and gastrointestinal disturbances.

Interactions

Drugs

Anticoagulants: theoretically, chondroitin could potentiate the effects of anticoagulants.

Dose

Not established. Doses of 200–400 mg two or three times a day (800–1200 mg daily) have been used, often combined with glucosamine.

References

1. Reginster JY, Heraud F, Zegels B, Bruyere O. Symptom and structure modifying properties of chondroitin sulfate in osteoarthritis. *Mini Rev Med Chem* 2007; 7: 1051–1061.

2. Uebelhart D, Knols R, de Bruin ED, Verbruggen G. Treatment of knee osteoarthritis with oral chondroitin sulfate. *Adv Pharmacol* 2006; 53: 523–539.

3. Lamari FN, Theocharis AD, Asimakopoulou AP, Malavaki CJ, Karamanos NK. Metabolism and biochemical/physiological roles of chondroitin sulfates: analysis of endogenous and supplemental chondroitin sulfates in blood circulation. *Biomed Chromatogr* 2006; 20: 539–550.

Chromium

Description

Chromium is a trace mineral found in two forms:

(1) trivalent (Cr^{3+}) which is biologically active and found in food
(2) hexavalent (Cr^{6+}), a toxic form that results from industrial pollution.

Human requirements

No UK reference nutrient intake (RNI) or estimated average requirement (EAR).

A safe and adequate intake is, for adults, 50–400 mcg daily; for children and adolescents, 0.1–1.0 mcg/kg daily.

US adequate intake (AI) for men (19–50 years) is 35 mcg daily and for women (19–50 years) 25 mcg daily. For those aged over 51, the AI is 30 mcg daily for men and 20 mcg daily for women.

Dietary sources

Wholegrain cereals (including bran cereals), brewers' yeast, broccoli, processed meats and spices are the best sources. Dairy products, most fruit and vegetables, and foods high in sugar are poor sources (diets high in simple sugars increase urinary chromium excretion compared with diets low in sugar, possibly because of increased chromium use in response to increased glucose metabolism).

Action

- Functions as an organic complex known as glucose tolerance factor (GTF).
- Enhances action of insulin.
- Influences carbohydrate, fat and protein metabolism.

Possible uses[1,2]

Health effect or disease risk	Strength of evidence
Helps control diabetes mellitus	P
Reduces cholesterol	I
Reduces body fat	P
Increases muscle/fat-free mass in athletes	I
Improves symptoms of depression associated with carbohydrate craving	P

I, insufficient; P, possible.

Bioavailability

Chromium picolinate seems to be better absorbed than chromium nicotinate and chromium chloride.[3]

Precautions/contraindications

Avoid taking chromium supplements containing yeast with monoamine oxidase inhibitors (MAOIs).

Pregnancy/breastfeeding

No problems reported at normal intakes.

Adverse effects

Trivalent chromium is relatively safe. There are reports of headaches, sleep disturbances and mood swings with chromium supplements. Chromium picolinate has been associated with genotoxicity and DNA damage, but this is not proven. Hexavalent chromium (not found in supplements) is toxic.

Interactions

Drugs

Antacids: may decrease chromium absorption.
Aspirin: may increase chromium absorption.

Insulin: may reduce insulin requirements in diabetes mellitus (monitor blood glucose).
Oral hypoglycaemics: may potentiate effects of oral hypoglycaemics.

Nutrients

Vitamin C: may increase chromium absorption.

Dose

Chromium is available in the form of chromium picolinate, chromium nicotinic acid, chromium chloride or as an organic complex in brewers' yeast.

The dose is not established. Studies have been conducted with 200–500 mcg elemental chromium daily. Dietary supplements provide, on average, 200 mcg in a daily dose.

References

1. Balk E, Tatsioni A, Lichtenstein A, Lau J, Pittas AG. Effect of chromium supplementation on glucose metabolism and lipids: a systematic review of randomized controlled trials. *Diabetes Care* 2007; 30: 2154–2163.
2. Vincent JB. The potential value and toxicity of chromium picolinate as a nutritional supplement, weight loss agent and muscle development agent. *Sports Med* 2003; 33: 213–230.
3. Disilvestro RA, Dy E. Comparison of acute absorption of commercially available chromium supplements. *J Trace Elem Med Biol* 2007; 21: 120–124.

Coenzyme Q10

Description

Coenzyme Q10 (ubiquinone) is a naturally occurring enzyme cofactor found in the mitochondria of the body cells. It is synthesised endogenously and intracellularly throughout body tissues, particularly the heart, liver, kidney and pancreas.

Human requirements

No proof of a dietary need exists. Carnitine is synthesised in sufficient quantities to meet human requirements.

Dietary sources

Meat and oily fish; smaller quantities in wholegrain cereals, soya beans, nuts and vegetables, particularly spinach and broccoli.

Action

- Involved in electron and proton transport.
- Supports the synthesis of adenosine triphosphate (ATP) in the mitochondrial membrane.
- Plays a vital role in intracellular energy production.
- Has antioxidant and immunostimulant activity.
- Helps to stabilise cell membranes, preserving cellular integrity and function.
- Helps to regenerate vitamin E to its antioxidant form.
- Essential for normal myocardial function.

Possible uses[1]

Health effect or disease risk	Strength of evidence
Improves symptoms of CVD	P

Improves symptoms of CHF	P
Improves symptoms of angina	P
Improves hypertension	P
Improves exercise performance	I
Improves symptoms of Parkinson's disease	I
Reduces breast cancer risk	I
Improves symptoms of migraine	I

I, insufficient; P, possible.

Bioavailability

Absorption of coenzyme Q10 is slow and limited. Solubilised formulations of coenzyme Q10 are superior to other forms (e.g. oily dispersions and crystalline Q10).[2,3]

Precautions/contraindications

Patients with CVD should seek medical advice before taking coenzyme Q10.

Caution when using high doses in patients on warfarin.

Pregnancy/breastfeeding

Safety not established.

Adverse effects

Doses up to 1200 mg/day have not been associated with adverse effects.[4] Gastrointestinal effects are reported rarely.

Interactions

Drugs

Statins: may deplete blood levels of coenzyme Q.
Warfarin: possible effects on international normalised ratio (INR).

Dose

Not established. Supplements provide doses of 10–150 mg/day.

References

1. Dhanasekaran M, Ren J. The emerging role of coenzyme Q-10 in aging, neurodegeneration, cardiovascular disease, cancer and diabetes mellitus. *Curr Neurovasc Res* 2005; 2: 447–459.

2. Bhagavan HN, Chopra RK. Plasma coenzyme Q10 response to oral ingestion of coenzyme Q10 formulations. *Mitochondrion* 2007; 7(suppl 1): S78–S88.

3. Schulz C, Obermuller-Jevic UC, Hasselwander O, Bernhardt J, Biesalski HK. Comparison of the relative bioavailability of different coenzyme Q10 formulations with a novel solubilizate (Solu Q10). *Int J Food Sci Nutr* 2006; 57: 546–555.

4. Hathcock JN, Shao A. Risk assessment for coenzyme Q10 (ubiquinone). *Regul Toxicol Pharmacol* 2006; 45: 282–288.

Conjugated linoleic acid

Description

Conjugated linoleic acid (CLA) is a class of conjugated isomers of the polyunsaturated fatty acid, linoleic acid. It contains two double bonds separated by a single bond. The main isomers identified in foods are *cis*-9, *trans*-10 (c9,t11)- and *trans*-10, *cis*-12 (t10,c12)-CLA. CLA is found in low concentrations in blood and other tissues, although it is not synthesised endogenously in humans. It is produced naturally by microorganisms associated with digestion, particularly in the rumen of cattle.

Human requirements

No proof of dietary need exists.

Dietary sources

Beef, lamb, dairy produce.

Action

- Antioxidant.
- Enhances immune function (in animals).
- Enhances delivery of fat into cells.
- Transports glucose into cells to provide energy and build muscle (rather than converting glucose to fat).

Possible uses[1–4]

Health effect or disease risk	Strength of evidence
Enhances weight loss	I
Reduces lean body bass and increases fat mass	P

continued

(continued)

Improves lipid profile	I
Improves insulin resistance	I
Reduces risk of cancer	I
Improves bone metabolism	I
Improves immune function	I

I, insufficient; P, possible.

Bioavailability

Biologically active CLA isomers are (c9,t11)-CLA and (t10,c12)-CLA. Several products contain the patented Clarinol or Tonalin formulas, which contain these isomers.

Precautions/contraindications

Insulin resistance.

Pregnancy/breastfeeding

No problems reported; insufficient data.

Adverse effects

No known adverse effects, except gastrointestinal effects, but no long-term studies. Lipid peroxidation reported in obese men with dose of 4.2 g/day; significance unknown.

Interactions

None reported.

Dose

Not established. Supplements provide 1–4 g/day.

References

1. Silveira MB, Carraro R, Monereo S, Tebar J. Conjugated linoleic acid (CLA) and obesity. *Public Health Nutr* 2007; 10(A): 1181–1186.

2. Hur SJ, Park Y. Effect of conjugated linoleic acid on bone formation and rheumatoid arthritis. *Eur J Pharmacol* 2007; 568: 16–24.
3. Salas-Salvado J, Marquez-Sandoval F, Bullo M. Conjugated linoleic acid intake in humans: a systematic review focusing on its effect on body composition, glucose, and lipid metabolism. *Crit Rev Food Sci Nutr* 2006; 46: 479–488.
4. Tricon S, Yaqoob P. Conjugated linoleic acid and human health: a critical evaluation of the evidence. *Curr Opin Clin Nutr Metab Care* 2006; 9: 105–110.

Copper

Description

Copper is an essential trace mineral.

Human requirements

DRVs for copper				
Age	UK		USA	
	RNI (mg/day)	EVM (mg/day)	Safe intake (mg/day)	TUL (mg/day)
0–3 months	0.3		0.2	–
4–6 months	0.3		0.22	–
7–12 months	0.3		0.22	–
1–3 years	0.4		0.34	1.0
4–6 years	0.6		1.0–1.5	–
4–8 years	–		0.44	3.0
7–10 years	0.7		–	–
9–13 years	–		0.7	5.0
14–18 years	–		0.89	8.0
Males				
11–14 years	0.8		–	–
15–18 years	1.0		–	–
19–50+ years	1.2	5	0.9	10.0
Females				
11–14 years	0.8		–	–
15–18 years	1.0		–	–
19–50+ years	1.2	5	0.9	10.0

Pregnancy	a		1.0	10.0[c]
Lactation	+0.3		1.0[b]	10.0[c]

EU RDA = none.
EAR, estimated average requirement; EU RDA, European Union recommended daily allowance; EVM, likely safe daily intake from supplements alone; LRNI, lower reference nutrient intake; RNI, reference nutrient intake; TUL, tolerable upper intake level.
[a]No increment.
[b]$\leq$18 years, 1.3 mg.
[c]$\leq$18 years, 8.0 mg.
Note: no EAR, LRNI or FAO/WHO RNIs have been derived for copper.

Dietary sources

Liver, shellfish, legumes, nuts, wholegrains.

Action

- Essential component of several enzymes, involved in various functions.
- Release of energy in the cytochrome system.
- Melanin production in the skin.
- Absorption and transport of iron.
- Formation of haemoglobin and transferrin.
- Production of catecholamine in the brain and adrenal gland.
- Metabolism of glucose, cholesterol and phospholipids.
- Synthesis of collagen and elastin.
- Detoxification of superoxide radicals.

Possible uses

Health effect or disease risk	Strength of evidence
Reduced serum cholesterol	I
Improved symptoms of arthritis	I
Improved symptoms of psoriasis	I

I, insufficient.

Bioavailability

No data from supplementation studies.

Precautions/contraindications

Avoid in Wilson's disease and biliary and hepatic impairment.

Pregnancy/breastfeeding

No problems with normal intakes.

Adverse effects

Excessive doses (not likely with supplements): epigastric pain, anorexia, nausea, vomiting and diarrhoea; hepatic toxicity and jaundice; hypotension; haematuria (blood in urine, pain on urination, lower back pain); metallic taste; convulsions and coma.

Interactions

Drugs

Penicillamine: reduces absorption of copper and vice versa; give 2 h apart.
Trientine: reduces absorption of copper and vice versa; give 2 h apart.

Nutrients

Iron: large doses of iron may reduce copper status and vice versa; give 2 h apart.
Vitamin C: large doses of vitamin C (>1 g daily) may reduce copper status.
Zinc: large doses of zinc may reduce absorption of copper and vice versa; give 2 h apart.

Dose

Copper supplements are available in the form of tablets and capsules, but mostly they are found in multivitamin and mineral supplements. The copper content of various commonly used salts is: copper amino acid chelate (20 mg/g); copper gluconate (140 mg/g); and copper sulphate (254 mg/g).

There is no established use or dose for copper as an isolated supplement.

Creatine

Description

Creatine is an amino acid synthesised from the amino acid precursors arginine, glycine and methionine. It is present in muscle, brain and blood. Trace amounts are also normally present in the urine.

Human requirements

No proof of a dietary need exists. Carnitine is synthesised in sufficient quantities to meet human requirements.

Dietary sources

Animal foods: fish and meat. Plant foods are poorer sources. The average omnivorous diet supplies about 1–2 g creatine daily.

Action

- Combines with phosphate to form creatine phosphate.
- As creatine phosphate, it acts as a source of high-energy phosphate and plays an essential part in the release of energy in muscle contraction.

Possible uses[1]

Health effect or disease risk	Strength of evidence
Increases the storage of creatine phosphate in muscle making more ATP available for working muscle	C
Increases muscle strength	P
Improves performance in single or repetitive high-intensity athletic activities	PR

continued

(*continued*)

Improves performance in prolonged submaximal exercise	I
Increases muscle strength in older people	P
Increases strength in heart failure	I
Increases strength in patients with muscular disorders	P

C, convincing; I, insufficient; P, possible; PR, probable.

Bioavailability

Maximal muscle storage of creatine is achieved with a dose of 5 g creatine monohydrate four times a day for 5–6 days, followed by 2 g daily to replace daily turnover.[2] Creatine administered in a solid form or as meat is readily absorbed but may result in slightly lower peak concentrations than the same dose ingested as a solution.[3]

Precautions/contraindications

Renal and hepatic impairment.

Pregnancy/breastfeeding

No problems reported but insufficient data.

Adverse effects

Nausea, diarrhoea, muscle cramps, dehydration reported.

Interactions

- No drug interactions.
- Caffeine may reduce or abolish the ergogenic effects of creatine.

Dose

Studies use 5 g four times a day for 5–6 days followed by 2 g daily. Do not exceed this dose.[4]

References

1. Brosnan JT, Brosnan ME. Creatine: endogenous metabolite, dietary, and therapeutic supplement. *Annu Rev Nutr* 2007; 27: 241–261.
2. Harris RC, Soderlund K, Hultman E. Elevation of creatine in resting and exercised muscle of normal subjects by creatine supplementation. *Clin Sci* 1992; 83: 367–374.
3. Harris RC, Nevill M, Harris DB, Fallowfield JL, Bogdanis GC, Wise JA. Absorption of creatine supplied as a drink, in meat or in solid form. *J Sports Sci* 2002; 20: 147–151.
4. Shao A, Hathcock JN. Risk assessment for creatine monohydrate. *Regul Toxicol Pharmacol* 2006; 45: 242–251.

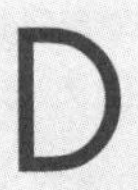

Dehydroepiandrosterone

Description

Dehydroepiandrosterone (DHEA) is an androgenic hormone produced in the adrenal glands. It is converted in the body to other hormones such as testosterone, oestrogen, progesterone and cortisol. DHEA levels peak between the ages of 20 and 30 years, then slowly decline.

Action

- A direct precursor to testosterone and oestrogen.
- Has oestrogenic and androgenic effects, the balance of which may depend on the individual's hormonal status.
- Stimulates insulin growth factor-1, which stimulates anabolism, insulin sensitivity and energy production, and accelerates muscle growth.

Possible uses[1,2]

Health effect or disease risk	Strength of evidence
Slows ageing	I
Enhances immunity	I
Helps weight loss	I
Improves insulin sensitivity	I
Enhances libido	I
Improves memory	I

continued

(continued)

Improves depression	I
Reduces symptoms of lupus	I
Beneficial for AIDS	I
Beneficial for cancer	I

I, insufficient.

Bioavailability

Administration of DHEA 50 mg/day or 100 mg/day to older men and women restored DHEA levels to the levels in young adults. Administration of 200 mg/day DHEA resulted in higher concentrations of DHEA in women than in men.[3]

Precautions/contraindications

Avoid in prostate cancer (or history of cancer), oestrogen-dependent cancer (e.g. breast or uterine cancer) or diabetes mellitus.

Pregnancy/breastfeeding

Avoid.

Adverse effects

No known toxicity, but no long-term safety data. Potential to increase oestrogenic and anabolic hormones; possible increase in risk of breast cancer and prostate cancer; in women, possible increased facial hair, increased loss of head hair, menstrual irregularities, deepening of voice.

Interactions

None reported. Theoretically interacts with insulin, oestrogens and androgens.

Dose

Not established; supplements provide 5–50 mg daily.

References

1. Morales AJ, Nolan JJ, Nelson JC *et al*. Effects of replacement dose of DHEA in men and women of advancing age. *J Clin Endocrinol Metab* 1994; 78: 1360–1367.

2. Morales AJ, Haubrich RH, Hwang JY, Asakura H, Yen SS. The effect of six months treatment with a 100 mg daily dose of dehydroepiandrosterone (DHEA) on circulating sex steroids, body composition and muscle strength in age-advanced men and women. *Clin Endocrinol (Oxf)* 1998; 49: 421–432.
3. Frye RF, Kroboth PD, Kroboth FJ *et al*. Sex differences in the pharmacokinetics of dehydroepiandrosterone (DHEA) after single- and multiple-dose administration in healthy older adults. *J Clin Pharmacol* 2000; 40: 596–605.

Dong quai

Description

Dong quai (*Angelica sinensis*) is a plant, the root of which is used in a dried form to produce food supplements.

Constituents

Ferulic acid, lingustilide, various vitamins and minerals, phytosterols, coumarin derivatives.

Action

Anticoagulant, anti-platelet, haematopoietic, antispasmodic, immunostimulatory, antioxidant and possibly oestrogenic activity.

Possible uses[1]

Health benefits	Evidence
Menopausal symptoms	I
Premenstrual syndrome (PMS)	I
Cardiovascular disease (treatment)	I

I, insufficient.

Precautions/contraindications

Avoid in hormone-sensitive conditions (breast, ovarian, endometrial cancer, endometriosis, uterine fibroids). Some constituents may be carcinogenic.

Pregnancy/breastfeeding

Avoid.

Adverse effects

No long-term safety data. May cause photosensitivity. Case report of gynaecomastia.

Interactions

Warfarin, anti-platelet drugs and anticoagulants: increased risk of bleeding.

Dose

Not established.

Reference

1. Monograph. *Angelica sinensis*. *Altern Med Rev* 2004; 9: 429–433.

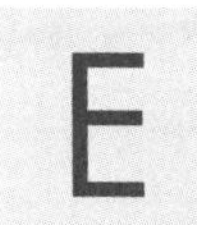

Evening primrose oil

Description

Evening primrose oil is derived from the seeds of *Oenothera biennis* and other species. It is synthesised endogenously from dietary linoleic acid (C18:2,*n*-6). Diabetes impairs this conversion.

Constituents

The oil content of the seeds is 17–25%, of which 8–11% is gamma-linolenic acid (GLA, C18:3,*n*-6).

Action

- Precursor of dihomogamma-linolenic acid (DGLA), series 1 prostaglandins (PG1s) and arachidonic acid.
- Activity of GLA is thought to be due to production of PG1s at expense of PG2s.
- PG1s have less inflammatory activity than PG2s.
- PGE_1 is a platelet aggregator and vasodilator.

Possible uses[1–4]

Health effect or disease risk	Strength of evidence
Improves eczema	P
Reduces symptoms of PMS	P
Reduces symptoms of rheumatoid arthritis	P

continued

(*continued*)

Improves diabetic neuropathy	P
Improves dry eye syndrome	I
Improves periodontal disease	I
Reduces risk of heart disease	I
Reduces risk of breast cancer	I
Improves asthma	I
Prevents hair loss	I

I, insufficient; P, possible.

Bioavailability

Acute administration of 280 mg GLA from 3 g of evening primrose oil resulted in a significant increase in plasma GLA concentrations in six volunteers. Maximum levels were reached in 2.7–4.4 hours.

Precautions/contraindications

Use of GLA has been associated with epilepsy and seizures. Recently, however, this has been questioned.[5]

Pregnancy/breastfeeding

Caution because of hormonal effects.

Adverse effects

Low toxicity. Nausea, diarrhoea and headache reported occasionally.

Interactions

Drugs

Phenothiazines: possibly increased risk of seizures, but this is now questioned.

Dose

Symptomatic relief of eczema: 320–480 mg (as GLA) daily; child aged 1–12 years, 160–320 mg daily.

Symptomatic relief of cyclical and non-cyclical mastalgia: 240–320 mg (as GLA) daily for 12 weeks (then stopped if no improvement).

Dietary supplements provide 40–300 mg (as GLA) per daily dose.

Note: doses are given in terms of GLA; evening primrose oil supplements are not identical; they provide different amounts of GLA.

References

1. Belch JJ, Hill A. Evening primrose oil and borage oil in rheumatologic conditions. *Am J Clin Nutr* 2000; 71(1 suppl): S352–S356.

2. Morse NL, Clough PM. A meta-analysis of randomized, placebo-controlled clinical trials of Efamol evening primrose oil in atopic eczema. Where do we go from here in light of more recent discoveries? *Curr Pharm Biotechnol* 2006; 7: 503–524.

3. Chenoy S, Hussain S, Tayob Y, O'Brien PMS, Moss MY, Morse PF. Effect of oral gamolenic acid from evening primrose oil on menopausal flushing. *BMJ* 1994; 308: 501–503.

4. Goyal A, Mansel RE. Efamast Study Group. A randomized multicenter study of gamolenic acid (Efamast) with and without antioxidant vitamins and minerals in the management of mastalgia. *Breast J* 2005; 11: 41–47.

5. Puri BK. The safety of evening primrose oil in epilepsy. *Prostaglandins Leukot Essent Fatty Acids* 2007; 77: 101–103.

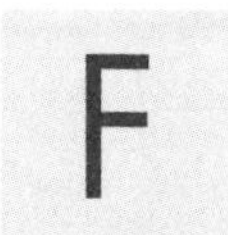

Fish oil

Description

There are two types of fish oil: fish liver oil (generally derived from the liver of the cod, halibut or shark) and fish body oil (generally derived from the flesh of the herring, sardine or anchovy).

Constituents

Both fish oil and fish liver oil are sources of omega-3 long-chain polyunsaturated fatty acids (LCPUFAs): eicosapentaenoic acid (EPA) and docosahexaenoic acid (DHA). They also contain vitamin E. Fish liver oil contains vitamin A (750–1200 mcg/daily dose) and vitamin D (2.5–10 mcg/daily dose).

Human requirements

Recommendations for intakes of omega-3 LCPUFAs	
Organisation	**Recommended intake**
UK Food Standards Agency (FSA)	Two portions of fish/week (including one oily); equivalent to 450 mg omega-3 LCPUFAs/day
British Dietetic Association	
People with heart disease	Two to three portions of high omega-3 (oily) fish/week *or* 0.5–1 g omega-3s (EPA and DHA) daily
Everyone else	Follow FSA recommendation
American Heart Association	
People without documented coronary heart disease (CHD)	Eat a variety of fish (preferably oily) at least twice a week

continued

(*continued*)

People with documented CHD People with raised triglycerides	1 g EPA/DHA daily preferably from fatty fish *or* consider supplement 1 g EPA + DHA/daily (with medical advice) 2–4 g/daily of EPA + DHA (with medical advice)
International Society for the Study of Fatty Acids and Lipids (ISSFAL)	Minimum of 500 mg/daily EPA + DHA for cardiovascular health
National Institute for Health and Clinical Excellence (NICE)	Post-myocardial infarction: 1 g daily LCPUFAs (preferably from oily fish, but from supplements if oily fish not consumed)
World Health Organization (WHO)	Two portions of fish/week; equivalent to 250–500 mg/daily EPA + DHA

EPA and DHA can also be synthesised in the body from alpha-linolenic acid (found in vegetables oils, e.g. soyabean, linseed and rapeseed oils, and nuts and seeds, e.g. walnuts, hemp and pumpkin), but conversion is poor (about 4%).

Dietary sources

Oily fish: mackerel, herring, kippers, pilchard, sardines, tuna, salmon.

Action

Fish oils have several effects, which are thought to result from a reduction in inflammatory and thrombotic prostaglandins, and leukotrienes and inflammatory cytokines. Effects include:

- Alteration of lipoprotein metabolism: reduced triglycerides; mixed effects on low- and high-density lipoprotein (LDL- and HDL)-cholesterol.
- Inhibition of atherosclerosis.
- Prevention of thrombosis.
- Reduction in heart rate.
- Influence of arrhythmias.
- Inhibition of inflammation.
- Inhibition of immune response.

Possible uses[1–9]

Health effect or disease risk	Strength of evidence
Cardiovascular disease:	
Reduced risk of CHD (primary)	PR
Reduced risk of CHD (secondary)	P
Reduced risk of stroke	P
Reduced mortality	PR

Lowers triglycerides Reduced blood clotting Inhibition of arrhythmia Lowers blood pressure Reduced angina	C C P C I
Arthritic conditions: Rheumatoid arthritis (management) Osteoarthritis (management)	 PR P
Inflammatory bowel disease: Crohn's disease (management) Ulcerative colitis (management)	 P P
Psoriasis (management)	I
Asthma (management)	I
Diabetes mellitus: Lowers triglycerides Glycaemic control	 C I
Cognitive health: Development of brain in infancy Dementia/Alzheimer's disease	 C P
Behavioural problems in children: Attention deficit hyperactivity disorder Developmental coordination disorder	 I P (improved reading, spelling, behaviour)
Visual acuity Infant visual acuity Reduced risk of age-related macular degeneration	 P P
Depression and mood disorders	I
Schizophrenia	I
Systemic lupus erythematosus	I
Cancer prevention	I

C, convincing; I, insufficient; P, possible; PR, probable.

Bioavailability

Supplements of fish oil and fish liver oil typically provide 100–2000 mg EPA + DHA per daily dose, sold as liquid oil or in softgel capsules. Studies have shown that concentrations of EPA and DHA in tissues,[10] chylomicrons[11] and serum[12] are increased in response to supplementation with pure oils.

Precautions/contraindications

- Monitor patients on anticoagulants (e.g. aspirin, warfarin).
- Stop supplementation before surgery.

- Vitamin A and D concentrations (if other supplements are taken concomitantly).
- Contaminants (e.g. dioxins, polychlorinated biphenyls); maximum contaminant level regulated by UK Committee on Toxicity (COT) and EU Scientific Committee on Food (SCF).

Pregnancy/breastfeeding

Avoid fish liver oils (vitamin A content).

Adverse effects

Possibly increased risk of bleeding (>3 g/day EPA + DHA).

Interactions

Anticoagulants (e.g. aspirin, warfarin): possibly increased risk of bleeding.
Bilberry, bromelain, dong quai, feverfew, flaxseed, garlic, ginger, gingko, ginseng, glucosamine, vitamin E: possibly increased risk of bleeding.

Dose

- See human requirements: follow recommendations for fish intake.
- If oily fish is not consumed:

  -healthy adults, EPA + DHA, up to 450 mg daily
  -people with cardiovascular disease, EPA + DHA, 0.5–1 g daily.

- Studies in arthritic conditions have used doses of EPA + DHA of 2–3 g daily. Studies in depression and other mental conditions have used doses of 1–10 g daily. Such doses should be used under medical supervision.

References

1. Simopoulos AP. Omega-3 fatty acids in inflammation and autoimmune diseases. *J Am Coll Nutr* 2002; 21: 495–505.
2. Wang C, Chung M, Balk E *et al. Effects of omega-3 fatty acids on cardiovascular disease.* Agency for Healthcare Research and Quality Evidence Report/ Technology Assessment: Number 94, 2004. Available from www.ahcpr.gov/ clinic/epcsums/o3cardsum.htm (accessed 30 October 2006).
3. Jacobson TA. Beyond lipids: the role of omega-3 fatty acids from fish oil in the prevention of coronary heart disease. *Curr Atheroscler Rep* 2007; 9: 145–153.
4. Yang H, Kenny A. The role of fish oil in hypertension. *Conn Med* 2007; 71: 533–538.

5. Turner D, Zlotkin SH, Shah PS, Griffiths AM. Omega 3 fatty acids (fish oil) for maintenance of remission in Crohn's disease. *Cochrane Database Syst Rev* 2007(2): CD006320.

6. DeLey M, deVos R, Hommes DW, Stokkers P. Fish oil for induction of remission in ulcerative colitis. *Cochrane Database Syst Rev* 2007(4): CD005986.

7. Turner D, Steinhart AH, Griffiths AM. Omega 3 fatty acids (fish oil) for maintenance of remission in ulcerative colitis. *Cochrane Database Syst Rev* 2007(3): CD006443.

8. Assisi A, Banzi R, Buonocore C *et al.* Fish oil and mental health: the role of n-3 long-chain polyunsaturated fatty acids in cognitive development and neurological disorders. *Int Clin Psychopharmacol* 2006; 21: 319–336.

9. Farmer A, Montori V, Dinneen S, Clar C. Fish oil in people with type 2 diabetes mellitus (Cochrane Review). *Cochrane Database Sys Rev* 2001(4): CD003205.

10. Arterburn LM, Hall EB, Oken H. Distribution, interconversion, and dose response of n-3 fatty acids in humans. *Am J Clin Nutr* 2006; 83(suppl): S1467–S1476.

11. Hansen JB, Grimsgaard S, Nilsen H, Nordoy A, Bonaa KH. Effects of highly purified eicosapentaenoic acid and docosahexaenoic acid on fatty acid absorption, incorporation into serum phospholipids and postprandial triglyceridemia. *Lipids* 1998; 33: 131–138.

12. Brox J, Olaussen K, Osterud B *et al.* A long-term seal- and cod-liver-oil supplementation in hypercholesterolemic subjects. *Lipids* 2001; 36: 7–13.

Flaxseed oil

Description

Flaxseed is the soluble fibre mucilage obtained from the fully developed seed of *Linus usitatissimum*.

Constituents

Alpha-linolenic acid and lignans. Alpha-linolenic acid is an essential fatty acid of the *n*-3 (omega-3) series, which can be converted into longer-chain fatty acids of the *n*-3 series, such as EPA and DHA. Conversion is limited.[1]

Action

- Source of omega-3 fatty acids.
- Omega-3 fatty acids are precursors to a range of prostaglandins, thromboxanes and leukotrienes, which are less proinflammatory than those of the *n*-6 series.

Possible uses[2–4]

Health effect or disease risk	Strength of evidence
Reduces cholesterol	I
Reduces risk of cardiovascular disease	P
Many help prevent cancer	I
Alleviates arthritis pain	I
Improves symptoms of eczema	I
Improves symptoms of psoriasis	I
Improves symptoms of lupus	I

I, insufficient; P, possible.

Bioavailability

Lack of significant data.

Precautions/contraindications

None.

Pregnancy/breastfeeding

No safety data.

Adverse effects

No known side effects or toxicity.

Interactions

None reported.

Dose

Not established.

References

1. Burdge GC, Calder PC. Conversion of alpha-linolenic acid to longer-chain polyunsaturated fatty acids in human adults. *Reprod Nutr Dev* 2005; 45: 581–597.

2. Wendland E. Farmer A, Glasziou P. Neil A. Effect of alpha linolenic acid on cardiovascular risk markers: a systematic review. *Heart* 2006; 92: 166–169.

3. Wilkinson P, Leach C, Ah-Sing EE *et al.* Influence of alpha-linolenic acid and fish-oil on markers of cardiovascular risk in subjects with an atherogenic lipoprotein profile. *Atherosclerosis* 2005; 181: 115–124.

4. Wang C, Harris WS, Chung M *et al.* n-3 Fatty acids from fish or fish-oil supplements, but not α-linolenic acid, benefit cardiovascular disease outcomes in primary- and secondary-prevention studies: a systematic review. *Am J Clin Nutr* 2006; 84: 5–17.

Fluoride

Description

Fluoride is a trace element.

Human requirements

No clear requirement for humans. No RNI has been set, but a safe and adequate intake, for infants only, is 0.05 mg/kg daily.

Dietary sources

Drinking water, tea, seafood.

Action

- Forms calcium fluoroapatite in teeth and bone.
- Protects against dental caries.
- May have a role in bone mineralisation.
- Helps remineralisation of bone in pathological conditions of demineralisation.

Possible uses[1]

Health effect or disease risk	Strength of evidence
Reduces risk of dental caries	C
Prevention of osteporosis	I
Prevention of fracture	I

C, convincing; I, insufficient.

Bioavailability

Lack of significant data.

Precautions/contraindications

Not for infants under 6 months and not in areas where the drinking water contains fluoride levels that exceed 700 mcg/L.

Pregnancy/breastfeeding

Insignificant data; best avoided.

Adverse effects

Chalky white patches on the surface of the teeth (may occur with recommended doses); yellow–brown staining of teeth, stiffness and aching of bones (with chronic excessive intake). Symptoms of acute overdose include diarrhoea, nausea, gastrointestinal cramp, bloody vomit, black stools, drowsiness, weakness, faintness, shallow breathing, tremors, and increased watering of mouth and eyes.

Interactions

None.

Dose

Refer first to fluoride content of water supply (contact local water board).

Daily doses[a] of fluoride (expressed as fluoride ion) in infants and children				
Fluoride content of water (mcg)	**Under 6 months**	**6 months–3 years (mcg)**	**3–6 years (mcg)**	**Over 6 years**
<300	None	250	500	1 mg
300–700	None	None	250	500 mcg
>700	None	None	None	None

[a]Recommended by the British Dental Association, the British Society of Paediatric Dentistry and the British Association for the Study of Community Dentistry.[2]

References

1. Smith GE. The action of fluoride in teeth and bone. *Med Hypotheses* 1986; 19: 139–154.
2. British Dental Association, the British Society of Paediatric Dentistry and the British Association for the Study of Community Dentistry. *Br Dent J* 1997; 182: 6–7.

Folic acid

Description

Folic acid is a water-soluble vitamin of the B complex.

Human requirements

DRVs for folic acid					
Age	UK		USA		FAO/WHO
	RNI (mcg/day)	EVM (mcg/day)	RDA (mcg/day)	TUL (mcg/day)	RNI (mcg/day)
0–3 months	50		65	–	80
4–6 months	50		65	–	80
7–12 months	50		80	–	80
1–3 years	70		150	300	150
4–6 years	100		–	–	200
4–8 years	–		200	400	–
7–10 years	150		–	–	300[a]
9–13 years	–		300	600	400
14–18 years	–		400	800	400
Males					
11–14 years	200		–	–	–
15–50+ years	200	1000	400	1000	400
Females					
11–14 years	200		–	–	–
15–50+ years	200	1000	400	1000	400

Pregnancy	+100[b]		600	1000[c]	600
Lactation	+60		500	1000[c]	600

EU RDA = 200 mcg.
EU RDA, European Union recommended daily allowance; EVM, likely safe daily intake from supplements alone; RDA, recommended daily allowance; RNI, reference nutrient intake; TUL, tolerable upper intake level.
[a]7–9 years
[b]The Department of Health recommends that all women who are pregnant or planning a pregnancy should take a folic acid supplement (see dose).
[c]≤ 18 years = 800 mcg daily.

Dietary sources

Wholegrain breakfast cereals, wholegrain bread, liver and kidney, green vegetables (e.g. Brussels sprouts, kale, spinach, broccoli), potatoes, pulses, oranges, yeast extract spreads.

Action

Lack of significant data.

Possible uses[1–9]

Health effect or disease risk	Strength of evidence
Reduced risk of neural tube defect	C
Cardiovascular disease: Reduces homocysteine Reduces risk of heart disease Reduced stroke	 PR P P
Reduces risk of cancer: Colon cancer Breast cancer Cervical cancer	P P I I
Mental disorders: Alzheimer's disease Depression	 I P

C, convincing; I, insufficient; P, possible; PR, probable.

Bioavailability

Supplements contain folic acid in the monoglutamate form, which requires no hydrolysis before absorption. This is in contrast to food folate, which is the polyglutamate form, and requires hydrolysis and removal of excess glutamates for absorption to occur.

1 mcg folic acid (on an empty stomach) = 1.2 mcg folic acid (with food) = 2 mcg food folate.[10]

Precautions/contraindications

Doses of folic acid > 400 mcg daily are not recommended if pernicious anaemia (vitamin B_{12} deficiency) is suspected.

Pregnancy/breastfeeding

No problems reported.

Adverse effects

Occasional gastrointestinal symptoms; allergy reported rarely.

Interactions

Drugs

Anticonvulsants: requirements for folic acid may be increased, but concurrent use of high-dose folic acid may antagonise the effects of anticonvulsants; an increase in anticonvulsant dose may be necessary in patients who receive supplementary folic acid (monitoring required).
Cholestyramine: may reduce the absorption of folic acid.
Methotrexate: acts as a folic acid antagonist; risk significant with high doses and/or prolonged use.
Oestrogens (including oral contraceptives): may reduce blood levels of folic acid.
Pyrimethamine: acts as a folic acid antagonist; risk significant with high doses and/or prolonged use; folic acid supplements should be given in pregnancy.
Sulfasalazine: may reduce the absorption of folic acid; requirements for folic acid may be increased.
Trimethoprim: acts as a folic acid antagonist; risk significant with high doses and/or prolonged use.
Zinc: high doses of folic acid may reduce absorption of zinc

Dose

- Prevention of first occurrence of neural tube defects (NTDs) in women who are planning a pregnancy: oral, 400 mcg daily before conception until week 12 of pregnancy.
-

Prevention of recurrence of NTDs: oral 5 mg daily before conception until week 12 of pregnancy.

- For prophylaxis during pregnancy (after week 12 if required to prevent deficiency), oral 200–500 mcg daily.
- In women with diabetes mellitus (increased risk of having a baby with a NTD), oral 5 mg daily before conception until week 12.[11]
- As a dietary supplement: oral, 100–500 mcg daily.
- When co-prescribed with methotrexate, in patients who suffer mucosal or gastrointestinal side effects with this drug, folic acid 5 mg each week may help to reduce the frequency of such side effects.[12]

References

1. Tamura T, Picciano MF. Folate and human reproduction. *Am J Clin Nutr* 2006; 83: 993–1016.
2. Goh YI, Koren G. Folic acid in pregnancy and fetal outcomes. *J Obstet Gynecol* 2008; 28: 3–13.
3. Wang X, Qin X, Demirtas H *et al*. Efficacy of folic acid supplementation in stroke prevention: a meta-analysis. *Lancet* 2007; 369: 1876–1882.
4. Bazzano LA, Reynolds K, Holder KN, He J. Effect of folic acid supplementation on risk of cardiovascular diseases: a meta-analysis of randomized controlled trials. *JAMA* 2006; 296: 2720–2726.
5. Carlsson CM. Homocysteine lowering with folic acid and vitamin B supplements: effects on cardiovascular disease in older adults. *Drugs Aging* 2006; 23: 491–502.
6. Strohle A, Wolters M, Hahn A. Folic acid and colorectal cancer prevention: molecular mechanisms and epidemiological evidence (Review). *Int J Oncol* 2005; 26: 1449–1464.
7. Coppen A, Bolander-Gouaille C. Treatment of depression: time to consider folic acid and vitamin B_{12}. *J Psychopharmacol* 2005; 19: 59–65.
8. Malouf R, Grimley Evans J, Areosa Sastre A. Folic acid with or without vitamin B_{12} for cognition and dementia. *Cochrane Database of Sys Rev* 2003 (4): CD004514.
9. Mischoulon D, Raab MF. The role of folate in depression and dementia. *J Clin Psychiatry* 2007; 68(suppl 10): 28–33.
10. Bailey LB. Dietary reference intakes for folate: the debut of dietary folate equivalents. *Nutr Rev* 1998; 56: 294–299.
11. www.clinicalanswers.nhs.uk/index.cfm?question=1473 (accessed 14 January 2006).
12. www.clinicalanswers.nhs.uk/index.cfm?question=248 (accessed 14 January 2006).

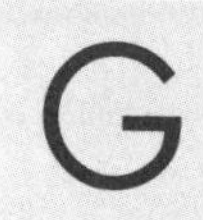

Gamma-oryzanol

Description

Gamma-oryzanol is one of several lipid fractions obtained from rice bran oil.

Constituents

Gamma-oryzanol is a mixture of phytosterols (plant sterols), including campesterol, cycloartanol, cycloartenol, beta-sitosterol, stigmasterol and ferulic acid.

Action

Phytosterols appear to reduce lipid levels and ferulic acid has antioxidant properties. Gamma-oryzanol has also been suggested to have anabolic properties, but evidence is conflicting.

Dietary sources

Brown rice, bran of cereals, fruit and vegetables.

Possible uses[1,2]

Health effect or disease risk	Strength of evidence
Lowers cholesterol	P
Improves exercise performance	I
Builds muscle	I
Reduces oxidative stress during exercise	I

I, insufficient; P, possible.

Bioavailability

No data.

Precautions/contraindications

None reported.

Pregnancy/breastfeeding

No problems reported but insufficient data.

Adverse effects

No long-term studies. Dry mouth, somnolence, hot flushes, irritability and headaches have been reported.

Interactions

None reported.

Dose

Not established. Dietary supplements provide 100–500 mg daily.

References

1. Cicero AF, Gaddi A. Rice bran oil and gamma-oryzanol in the treatment of hyperlipoproteinaemias and other conditions. *Phytother Res* 2001; 15: 277–289.
2. Fry AC, Bonner E, Lewis DL *et al*. The effects of gamma-oryzanol supplementation during resistance exercise training. *Int J Sport Nutr* 1997; 7: 318–329.

Garlic

Description

Garlic is the fresh bulb of *Allium sativum*, which is related to the lily family (Liliaceae).

Constituents

The major active constituents of garlic include alliin, allicin, diallyl disulphide, *S*-allyl cysteine and ajoene. Crushing or chopping garlic releases allinase which catalyses the formation of allicin. Crushing raw garlic and then allowing it to sit for 10 minutes helps retain some of the biologically active constituents that are destroyed during cooking. Allicin appears to be one of the most pharmacologically active constituents in relation to cholesterol lowering.

Dietary sources

Allium vegetables, including garlic and onions, are the richest source of organosulphur compounds in the human diet.

Human requirements

No requirement for garlic, but one clove daily may be beneficial.

Action

- Antioxidant.
- Inhibits platelet aggregation.
- Antithrombotic.
- Stimulates fibrinolysis.
- Reduces serum cholesterol.
- Antihypertensive.
- Antimicrobial.
- Enhancement of immune function.
- Antineoplastic activity.

- Anti-inflammatory.
- Hypoglycaemic.

Possible uses[1–5]

Health effect or disease risk	Strength of evidence
Reduces cholesterol	PR
Controls blood pressure	PR
Improves circulation	P
Improves walking distance in peripheral arterial disease	I
Reduced risk of cancer	I
Antifungal, antiviral, antibacterial activity	I

I, insufficient; P, possible; PR, probable.

Bioavailability

Fresh garlic cloves contain 6–14 mg/g of alliin. Garlic cloves yield about 2500–4500 mcg of allicin per gram of fresh weight when crushed. One clove of garlic weighs 2–4 g.

Precautions/contraindications

Hypersensitivity to garlic.

Pregnancy/breastfeeding

No problems reported, but insufficient study data.

Adverse effects

Unpleasant breath odour, indigestion, gastrointestinal irritation; sensitivity reactions (e.g. dermatitis, asthma).

Interactions

None reported. Theoretically, garlic could increase bleeding with blood-thinning drugs (e.g. aspirin, warfarin) or supplements (e.g. bromelain, dong quai, fish oil, flaxseed, ginger, ginkgo, vitamin E).

Dose

Not established, but 400–1000 mg (equivalent to 2–5 g fresh garlic or one to two cloves) daily of a standardised garlic product has been used in several studies. Dietary supplements provide 400–1000 mg dried garlic daily. Standardised products may be standardised for allicin potential. However, allicin is now known not to be the only important active ingredient in garlic. One clove of fresh garlic is equivalent to 4000 mcg allicin potential.

References

1. Gorinstein S, Jastrzebski Z, Namiesnik J, Leontowicz H, Leontowicz M, Trakhtenberg S. The atherosclerotic heart disease and protecting properties of garlic: contemporary data. *Mol Nutr Food Res* 2007; 51: 1365–1381.
2. Ngo SN, Williams DB, Cobiac L, Head RJ. Does garlic reduce risk of colorectal cancer? A systematic review. *J Nutr* 2007; 137: 2264–2269.
3. Borek C. Garlic reduces dementia and heart-disease risk. *J Nutr* 2006; 136 (suppl): S810–S812.
4. Rahman K, Lowe GM. Garlic and cardiovascular disease: a critical review. *J Nutr* 2006; 136(suppl): S736–S740.
5. Harris JC, Cottrell SL, Plummer S, Lloyd D. Antimicrobial properties of *Allium sativum* (garlic). *Appl Microbiol Biotechnol* 2001; 57: 282–286.

Ginkgo biloba

Description

Ginkgo biloba is an extract from the dried leaves of *Ginkgo biloba* (maidenhair tree).

Constituents

The leaf contains amino acids, flavonoids and terpenoids (including bilobalide and ginkgolides A, B, C, J and M).

Action

- Stimulates prostaglandin biosynthesis.
- Vasoregulatory effects on catecholamines.
- Antagonises platelet-activating factor (PAF), reducing platelet aggregation and decreasing the production of oxygen free radicals.
- Increases blood flow, produces arterial vasodilatation and reduces blood viscosity.
- Free radical scavenger and antioxidant.
- May influence neurotransmitter metabolism.

Possible uses[1–5]

Health effect or disease risk	Strength of evidence
Improves memory (in Alzheimer's disease)	P
Improves memory and concentration in healthy people	P
Improves circulation and walking in peripheral vascular disease	P
Improves tinnitus	I
Altitude (mountain) sickness	I
Depression and seasonal affective disorder	I
Glaucoma	I

Age-related macular degeneration	I
Benefit in multiple sclerosis	I
Benefit in premenstrual syndrome	I
Benefit in vertigo	I

I, insufficient; P, possible.

Bioavailability

Oral gingko biloba has been shown to be 60% absorbed in rat studies.[6] In humans a dose of 40 mg twice daily demonstrates better bioavailability than a dose of 80 mg daily.[7]

Precautions/contraindications

Avoid in hypertension, bleeding disorders,[8] epilepsy. Monitor blood glucose in diabetes.

Pregnancy/breastfeeding

Contraindicated in pregnant[9] and breastfeeding women, and in children.

Adverse effects

Headache, nausea, vomiting, heartburn and diarrhoea have been reported occasionally. There have been rare reports of severe allergic reactions, including skin reactions (e.g. itching, erythema and blisters) and convulsions.

Interactions[10]

May increase bleeding with blood-thinning drugs (e.g. aspirin, warfarin) or supplements (e.g. bromelain, dong quai, fish oil, flaxseed, ginger, ginkgo, vitamin E).

Dose

Most clinical trials have used a 50:1 concentrated leaf extract (EGb 761) standardised to 24% flavone glycosides and 6% terpene glycones. (A standardised 40 mg tablet should therefore contain 9.6 mg flavone glycosides and 2.4 mg terpene glycones.) Studies have used 120–240 mg daily. Dietary supplements provide 40–80 mg in a dose.

References

1. Ramassamy C, Longpre F, Christen Y. Ginkgo biloba extract (EGb 761) in Alzheimer's disease: is there any evidence? *Curr Alzheimer Res* 2007; 4: 253–262.

2. Birks J, Grimley Evans J. *Ginkgo biloba* for cognitive impairment and dementia. *Cochrane Database Syst Rev* 2002(4): CD003120.

3. Smith PF, Zheng Y, Darlington CL. *Ginkgo biloba* extracts for tinnitus: more hype than hope? *J Ethnopharmacol* 2005; 100: 95–99.

4. Zhou W, Chai H, Lin PH, Lumsden AB, Yao Q, Chen C. Clinical use and molecular mechanisms of action of extract of *Ginkgo biloba* leaves in cardiovascular diseases. *Cardiovasc Drug Rev* 2004; 22: 309–319.

5. Horsch S, Walther C. Ginkgo biloba special extract EGb 761 in the treatment of peripheral arterial occlusive disease (PAOD) – a review based on randomized, controlled studies. *Int J Clin Pharmacol Ther* 2004; 42: 63–72.

6. Moreau JP, Eck CR, McCabe J, Skinner S. [Absorption, distribution and elimination of a labelled extract of *Ginkgo biloba* leaves in the rat]. *Presse Med* 1986; 15: 1458–1461.

7. Drago F, Floriddia ML, Cro M, Giuffrida S. Pharmacokinetics and bioavailability of a *Ginkgo biloba* extract. *J Ocul Pharmacol Ther* 2002; 18: 197–202.

8. Bent S, Goldberg H, Padula A, Avins AL. Spontaneous bleeding associated with ginkgo biloba: a case report and systematic review of the literature. *J Gen Intern Med* 2005; 20: 657–661.

9. Dugoua JJ, Mills E, Perri D, Koren G. Safety and efficacy of ginkgo (*Ginkgo biloba*) during pregnancy and lactation. *Can J Clin Pharmacol* 2006; 13: e277–e284.

10. Bressler R. Herb–drug interactions: interactions between *Ginkgo biloba* and prescription medications. *Geriatrics* 2005; 60(4): 30–33.

Ginseng

Description

Ginseng is the collective term used to describe several species of plants belonging to the genus *Panax*. These include the Asian ginsengs (*Panax ginseng* and *Panax japonicus*) and American ginseng (*Panax quinquefolius* L). Siberian/Russian ginseng (*Eleuthrococcus senticosus*) is not considered to be true ginseng because it is not a species of the genus *Panax*.

Constituents

Triterpene saponins (ginsenosides), essential oil-containing polyacetylenes and sesquiterpenes, polysaccharides, peptidoglycans and nitrogen-containing compounds.

Action

- Analgesic.
- Antipyretic.
- Anti-inflammatory.
- Central nervous system (CNS)-stimulating and CNS-depressant activity.
- Hypotensive and hypertensive activity.
- Histamine-like activity and antihistamine activity.
- Hypoglycaemic activity.
- Erythropoietic activity.
- Interacts with central cholinergic and dopaminergic pathways.

Possible uses[1–5]

Health effect or disease risk	Strength of evidence
Improves exercise performance (boost energy)	P
Improves mental performance (boosts mood)	P
Adaptogen (helps normalise imbalances in disease states)	I

continued

(*continued*)

Helps control blood sugar in diabetes	P
Prevents cancer	I
Improves heart function in CHD and CHF	I
Reduces blood pressure	I
Erectile dysfunction	I
Prevents upper respiratory tract infection	I
Enhances immune system	I
Relieves menopausal symptoms	I
Improves sense of well-being	I

I, insufficient; P, possible.

Precautions/contraindications

Avoid in children. Caution in cardiovascular disease, diabetes mellitus, asthma, schizophrenia and CNS disorders.

Pregnancy/breastfeeding

Avoid.

Adverse effects[6]

Insomnia, nervous excitation, euphoria; nausea and diarrhoea (especially in the morning); skin eruptions; oedema; oestrogenic effects (e.g. breast tenderness; temporary return of menstruation in postmenopausal women).

Interactions[6]

Drugs

Tranquillisers: ginseng may reverse the effects of sedatives and tranquillisers.
Digoxin: ginseng may increase blood levels of digoxin.
Warfarin: ginseng may influence the effect of warfarin.

Dose

Not established. Manufacturers tend to recommend 0.5–3 g daily of the dried root or its equivalent.

References

1. Buettner C, Yeh GY, Phillips RS *et al*. Systematic review of the effects of ginseng on cardiovascular risk factors. *Ann Pharmacother* 2006; 40: 83–95.
2. Xie JT, McHendale S, Yuan CS. Ginseng and diabetes. *Am J Chin Med* 2005; 33: 397–404.
3. Kaneko H, Nakanishi K. Proof of the mysterious efficacy of ginseng: basic and clinical trials: clinical effects of medical ginseng, Korean red ginseng: specifically, its anti-stress action for prevention of disease. *J Pharmacol Sci* 2004; 95: 158–162.
4. Coleman CI, Hebert JH, Reddy P. The effects of *Panax ginseng* on quality of life. *J Clin Pharm Ther* 2003; 28: 5–15.
5. Kennedy DO, Scholey AB. Ginseng: potential for the enhancement of cognitive performance and mood. *Pharmacol Biochem Behav* 2003; 75: 687–700.
6. Coon JT, Ernst E. *Panax ginseng:* a systematic review of adverse effects and drug interactions. *Drug Safety* 2002; 25: 323–344.

Glucosamine

Description

Glucosamine is a natural substance found in mucopolysaccharides, mucoproteins and chitin. Naturally present in cartilage with other substances.

Constituents

It is a hexosamine sugar (compound of glucose and an amine).

Dietary sources

Crabs, oysters, shells of prawns. (However, supplements are the most effective source of additional glucosamine.)

Action

- A basic building block for the biosynthesis of glycoprotein, glycolipids, hyaluronic acid, glycosaminoglycans and proteoglycans, which are important constituents of articular cartilage.
- Important for maintaining the elasticity, strength and resilience of cartilage in joints.
- Helps to reduce damage to the joints.
- Enhances the production of hyaluronic acid and its anti-inflammatory action.

Possible uses[1,2]

Health effect or disease risk	Strength of evidence
Relieves knee osteoarthritis	C
Relieves osteoarthritis (general)	PR
Relieves rheumatoid arthritis	I
Helps damage to tendons and ligaments from sports injuries	I

Improves symptoms of tendonitis and bursitis	I
Improves inflammatory bowel disease	I
Improves chronic venous insufficiency	I

C, convincing; I, insufficient; PR, probable.

Bioavailability

Oral glucosamine has been shown to be 90% absorbed and diffused into bone and articular cartilage.[3] Two further studies[4,5] with oral crystalline glucosamine sulphate found that glucosamine from this formulation is bioavailable both systemically and at the site of action.

Precautions/contraindications

Caution in diabetes mellitus. Mixed findings on glucose metabolism.[6,7] Monitor carefully.

Pregnancy/breastfeeding

No problems reported but insufficient data; probably best avoided.

Adverse effects

Constipation, diarrhoea, heartburn, nausea, drowsiness, headache and rash reported occasionally.

Interactions

None reported. In theory, anti-diabetic drugs and insulin may be less effective.

Dose

Usual dose, 500 mg three times a day.

References

1. Bruyere O, Pavelka K, Rovati LC *et al*. Glucosamine sulfate reduces osteoarthritis progression in postmenopausal women with knee osteoarthritis: evidence from two 3-year studies. *Menopause* 2004; 11: 134–135.
2. Vlad SC, LaValley MP, McAlindon TE, Felson DT. Glucosamine for pain in osteoarthritis: why do trial results differ? *Arthritis Rheum* 2007; 56: 2267–2277.

3. Setnikar I, Palumbo R, Canali S, Zanolo G. Pharmacokinetics of glucosamine in man. *Arzneimittelforschung* 1993; 43: 1109–1113.
4. Persiani S, Roda E, Rovati LC, Locatelli M, Giacovelli G, Roda A. Glucosamine oral bioavailability and plasma pharmacokinetics after increasing doses of crystalline glucosamine sulfate in man. *Osteoarthritis Cartilage* 2005; 13: 1041–1049.
5. Persiani S, Rotini R, Trisolino G *et al.* Synovial and plasma glucosamine concentrations in osteoarthritic patients following oral crystalline glucosamine sulphate at therapeutic dose. *Osteoarthritis Cartilage* 2007; 15: 764–772.
6. Marshall PD, Poddar S, Tweed EM, Brandes L. Clinical inquiries: Do glucosamine and chondroitin worsen blood sugar control in diabetes? *J Fam Pract* 2006; 55: 1091–1093.
7. Stumpf JL, Lin SW. Effect of glucosamine on glucose control. *Ann Pharmacother* 2006; 40: 694–698.

Grape seed extract

Description

Grape seed extract is an extract from the tiny seeds of red grapes.

Constituents

Oligomeric proanthocyanidin complexes (proanthocyanidins), a category of flavonoids derived from flavan-3-ols and flavan-3,4-diols, made up of dimers or trimers of catechin and epicatechin. Also includes essential fatty acids and tocopherols.

Action

- Antioxidant: neutralises free radicals, including hydroxyl groups and lipid peroxides, blocking lipid peroxidation and stabilising cell membranes.
- Inhibits destruction of collagen by stabilising the activity of α_1-antitrypsin, which inhibits the activity of substances such as elastin and hyaluronic acid (this is thought to prevent fluid exudation by allowing red blood cells to cross the capillaries).
- Inhibits the release of inflammatory mediators, such as histamine and prostaglandins.
- Inhibits platelet aggregation.
- Antibacterial, antiviral and anti-carcinogenic activity.

Possible uses[1]

Health effect or disease risk	Strength of evidence
Maintains healthy lipid profile	I
Improves symptoms of venous insufficiency	P
Improves poor capillary resistance	P
Reduces oxidative stress	P
Treatment of seasonal allergic rhinitis	I

I, insufficient; P, possible.

Bioavailability

The bioavailability of grape seed constituents in humans and animals is unclear.

Precautions/contraindications

None known.

Pregnancy/breastfeeding

No problems reported, but insufficient study data.

Adverse effects

None reported, but no long-term safety data.

Interactions

None reported, but in theory bleeding tendency may be increased with anti-coagulants, aspirin and anti-platelet drugs.

Dose

Not established. Doses of 100–300 mg (standardised to contain 92–95% proanthocyanidins) have been used in studies.

Reference

1. Bagchi D, Sen CK, Ray SD *et al.* Molecular mechanisms of cardioprotection by a novel grape seed proanthocyanidin extract. *Mutat Res* 2003; 523–524: 87–97.

Green-lipped mussel

Description

Green-lipped mussel extract comes from *Perna canaliculata*, a salt-water shellfish indigenous to New Zealand.

Constituents

May contain a prostaglandin inhibitor that is anti-inflammatory (possibly omega-3 fatty acid). Contains about 2% lipids: phospholipids, triglycerides, free fatty acids (polyunsaturated fatty acids, monounsaturated fatty acids, saturated fatty acids, triglycerides).

Action

Anti-inflammatory activity.

Possible uses[1]

Health effect or disease risk	Strength of evidence
Improves symptoms in rheumatoid arthritis	I
Improves symptoms in osteoarthritis	I
Improves symptoms in asthma	I

I, insufficient.

Bioavailability

No data.

Precautions/contraindications

None.

Pregnancy/breastfeeding

No problems reported, but no safety data in pregnant women.

Adverse effects

Diarrhoea, nausea, flatulence.

Interactions

None reported.

Dose

Not established. Supplements provide 1 g/daily dose.

Reference

1. Brien S, Prescott P, Coghlan B, Bashir N, Lewith G. Systematic review of the nutritional supplement *Perna canaliculus* (green-lipped mussel) in the treatment of osteoarthritis. *Q J Med* 2008; 101: 167–179.

Green tea extract

Description

A non-fermented product (black tea is fermented) made from the leaves of *Camellia sinensis*.

Constituents

Green tea catechins (potent polyphenolic antioxidants with a flavan-3-olic structure). They include seven types: (–)-gallocatechin (GC), (–)-epigallocatechin (EGC), (+)-catechin (C), (–)-epigallocatechin-3-gallate (EGCG), (–)-epicatechin (EC), (–)-gallocatechingallate (GCG) and (–)-epicatechingallate (ECG). Also contains flavonols, tannins, minerals, free amino acids and methylxanthines (caffeine, theophylline and theobromine).

Action

- Antioxidant.
- Chemoprotective.
- Antibacterial and antiviral activity.
- Reduction of serum cholesterol and LDL-cholesterol oxidation.
- Inhibition of platelet aggregation.

Possible uses[1–5]

Health effect or disease risk	Strength of evidence
Antioxidant/reduces oxidative stress	PR
Reduces risk of cancer	P
Reduces serum cholesterol	I
Reduces risk of heart disease	I
Reduces body weight	I
Improves insulin resistance	I

continued

(continued)

Improves cognitive function	I
Improves menopausal symptoms	I
Benefits in asthma	I
Reduces inflammation in arthritis	I

I, insufficient; P, possible; PR, probable.

Bioavailability

EGCG, EGC and EC have been shown in plasma following consumption of green tea.[6,7]

Precautions/contraindications

None.

Pregnancy/breastfeeding

No problems reported but insufficient study data.

Adverse effects

Insufficient data with green tea extracts. Case reports of liver toxicity with extracts (may be caused by contaminants).

Interactions

None reported. Theoretically, green tea extract could increase bleeding with blood-thinning drugs (e.g. aspirin, warfarin) or supplements (e.g. bromelain, dong quai, fish oil, flaxseed, ginger, ginkgo, vitamin E).

Dose

Not established, but doses of 250–300 mg daily have been used. Supplements should be standardised (and labelled) to contain 50–97% polyphenols, containing per dose at least 50% (–)-epigallocatechin-3-gallate. Four to six cups of freshly brewed green tea should provide similar levels of polyphenols.

References

1. Wolfram S. Effects of green tea and EGCG on cardiovascular and metabolic health. *J Am Coll Nutr* 2007; 26: S373–S388.

2. Chen L, Zhang HY. Cancer preventive mechanisms of the green tea polyphenol (−)-epigallocatechin-3-gallate. *Molecules* 2007; 12: 946–957.
3. Basu A, Lucas EA. Mechanisms and effects of green tea on cardiovascular health. *Nutr Rev* 2007; 65(8 Pt 1): 361–375.
4. Cabrera C, Artacho R, Gimenez R. Beneficial effects of green tea – a review. *J Am Coll Nutr* 2006; 25: 79–99.
5. Wolfram S, Wang Y, Thielecke F. Anti-obesity effects of green tea: from bedside to bench. *Mol Nutr Food Res* 2006; 50: 176–187.
6. Yang CS, Chen L, Lee MJ, Balentine D, Kuo MC, Schantz SP. Blood and urine levels of tea catechins after ingestion of different amounts of green tea by human volunteers. *Cancer Epidemiol Biomarkers Prev* 1998; 7: 351–354.
7. Lee MJ, Maliakal P, Chen L *et al.* Pharmacokinetics of tea catechins after ingestion of green tea and (−)-epigallocatechin-3-gallate by humans: formation of different metabolites and individual variability. *Cancer Epidemiol Biomarkers Prev* 2002; 11(10 Pt 1): 1025–1032.

Guarana

Description

Guarana is produced from the dried and powdered seeds of a South American shrub, *Paullinia cupana*.

Constituents

Guaranine (a synonym for caffeine); theobromine, theophylline and tannins.

Action

- A CNS stimulant.
- Increases heart rate and contractility.
- Increases blood pressure.
- Inhibits platelet aggregation.
- Stimulates gastric acid secretion.
- Diuretic.
- Relaxes bronchial smooth muscle.
- Stimulates the release of catecholamines.

Possible uses[1,2]

Health effect or disease risk	Strength of evidence
Improves mental alertness	PR
Improves stamina and endurance in athletes	P
Improves immunity	I
Retards ageing	I
Appetite suppressant	I
Alleviates migraine	I
Alleviates anxiety and tension	I
Alleviates constipation	I

I, insufficient; P, possible; PR, probable.

Bioavailability

No data.

Precautions/contraindications

Avoid in cardiovascular disease, peptic ulcer, anxiety disorders and renal impairment. It should also not be taken within 2 h of bedtime.

Pregnancy/breastfeeding

Avoid.

Adverse effects

High doses of guarana may cause insomnia, nervousness, irritability, palpitations, gastric irritation, flushing and elevated blood pressure.

Interactions

None reported.

Dose

Not established. Dietary supplements provide 50–200 mg/dose.

References

1. Kennedy DO, Haskell CF, Wesnes KA, Scholey AB. Improved cognitive performance in human volunteers following administration of guarana (*Paullinia cupana*) extract: comparison and interaction with *Panax ginseng*. *Pharmacol Biochem Behav* 2004; 79: 401–411.
2. Haskell CF, Kennedy DO, Wesnes KA, Milne AL, Scholey AB. A double-blind, placebo-controlled, multi-dose evaluation of the acute behavioural effects of guarana in humans. *J Psychopharmacol* 2007; 21: 65–70.

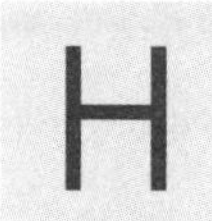

Hydroxycitric acid

Description

Hydroxycitric acid (HCA) is derived from the small fruit of the plant *Garcinia cambogia* found in south-east Asia.

Action

HCA is a potent inhibitor of the enzyme ATP citrate lyase. Inhibition of ATP citrate lyase has the capacity to prevent carbohydrate conversion to fat. Inhibition of this conversion may suppress appetite and inhibit adipose tissue synthesis.

Possible uses[1]

Health effect or disease risk	Strength of evidence
Reduces body weight[a]	I
Reduces appetite	I
Improves lipid profile	I

[a]Improved evidence in preparation of increased bioavailability.[2]
I, insufficient.

Precautions/contraindications

No long-term studies have assessed the safety of HCA.

Pregnancy/breastfeeding

No data in pregnant/breastfeeding women. HCA is best avoided during pregnancy and lactation.

Adverse effects

No serious side effects have been noted.

Interactions

None reported.

Dose

Not established. Manufacturers recommend taking 250–1500 mg daily of HCA.

References

1. Jena BS, Jayaprakasha GK, Singh RP, Sakariah KK. Chemistry and biochemistry of (–)-hydroxycitric acid from *Garcinia*. *J Agric Food Chem* 2002; 50: 10–22.

2. Preuss HG, Garis RI, Bramble JD *et al*. Efficacy of a novel calcium/potassium salt of (–)-hydroxycitric acid in weight control. *Int J Clin Pharmacol Res* 2005; 25: 133–144.

5-Hydroxytryptophan

Description

An amino acid precursor of serotonin. Supplements of 5-hydroxytryptophan (5HTP) were banned in the UK in 1990 as a result of the association with eosinophilic myalgia syndrome (EMS) and several fatalities. After the suggestion that contaminants (not 5HTP) could be the cause, supplements have been available since 2001.

Action

HCA may raise brain serotonin levels (possibly beneficial effects on disorders associated with low serotonin levels, e.g. anxiety, depression, aggression, insomnia, pain sensation and sexual behaviour).[1]

Possible uses[2–4]

Health benefits	Evidence
Depression	P
Anxiety	I
Insomnia	I
Fibromyalgia	I
Headache	I
Weight reduction	I

I, insufficient; P, possible.

Bioavailability

Oral bioavailability: 47–84% (mean 69.2%).

Precautions/contraindications

Controversial. Associated with EMS. May be caused by contaminants. Insufficient evidence as to whether EMS is caused by 5HTP or contaminant.[5,6]

Pregnancy/breastfeeding

Avoid.

Adverse effects

Possibly EMS (see above); gastrointestinal disturbances (nausea, heartburn, flatulence, satiety); high doses: serotonin syndrome (euphoria, drowsiness, hyperreactivity of reflexes, sustained rapid eye movement [REM], rapid muscle contraction and abnormal movement of ankle and jaw, high temperature, sweating, muscle twitching, feeling drunk, dizziness, clumsiness, restlessness).

Interactions

Drugs

Antidepressants (selective serotonin release inhibitors [SSRIs], monoamine oxidase inhibitors [MAOIs], trazodone, venlafaxine): may be synergistic with 5HTP.
Carbidopa: associated with scleroderma (hard, thick, inflamed skin) with 5HTP.
Sumatriptan: may increase serotonin levels.
Tramodol: may increase serotonin levels.
Zolpidem: theoretically could cause hallucinations with 5HTP.

Dose

Not established. Best avoided until clear evidence of safety.

References

1. Birdsall TC. 5-Hydroxytryptophan: a clinically-effective serotonin precursor. *Altern Med Rev* 1998; 3: 271–280.
2. Shaw K, Turner J, Del Mar C. Tryptophan and 5-hydroxytryptophan for depression. *Cochrane Database Syst Rev* 2002(1): CD003198.
3. Dayan P, Huys QJ. Serotonin, inhibition, and negative mood. *PLoS Comput Biol* 2008; 4(2): e4.
4. Byerley WF, Judd LL, Reimherr FW, Grosser BI. 5-Hydroxytryptophan: a review of its antidepressant efficacy and adverse effects. *J Clin Psychopharmacol* 1987; 7: 127–137.

5. Food and Drug Administration. FDA Talk Paper. Impurities confirmed in dietary supplement 5-hydroxytryptophan. Rockville, MD: FDA, 1998. Available at http://vm.cfsan.fda.gov/~lrd/tp5htp.html (accessed 29 February 2008).

6. Michelson D, Page SW, Casey R *et al*. An eosinophilia–myalgia syndrome related disorder associated with exposure to L-5-hydroxytryptophan. *J Rheumatol* 1994; 21: 2261–2265.

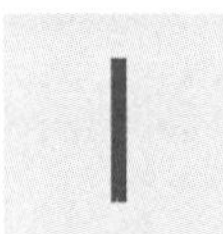

Iodine

Description

Iodine is an essential trace element.

Human requirements

DRVs for iodine						
Age	UK			USA		WHO/ FAO
	LNRI (mcg/ day)	RNI (mcg/ day)	EVM (mcg/ day)	RDA (mcg/ day)	TUL (mcg/ day)	RNI (mcg/ day)
0–3 months	40	50		110[b]	–	90
4–6 months	40	60		110[b]	–	90
7–12 months	40	60		130	–	90
1–3 years	40	70		90	200	90
4–6 years	50	100		–	–	–
4–8 years	–	–		90	300	
7–10 years	55	110		–	–	120[c]
9–13 years	–	–		120	600	–
14–18 years	–	–		150	900	150[d]

continued

(continued)

Males and females						
11–14 years	65	130		–	–	–
15–18 years	70	140		–	–	–
19–50+	70	140	500	150	1100	150
Pregnancy	[a]	[a]		220	1100	200
Lactation	[a]	[a]		290	1100	200

EU RDA = 150 mcg.
EU RDA, European Union recommended daily allowance; EVM, likely safe daily intake from supplements alone; LNRI, lower reference nutrient intake; RDA, recommended daily allowance; RNI, reference nutrient intake; TUL, tolerable upper intake level.
[a]No increment.
[b]Adequate intakes (AIs).
[c]6–12 years.
[d]13–18 years.

Dietary intake

In the UK, the average adult diet provides: for men, 220 mcg daily; for women, 159 mcg daily.

Action

Iodine is an essential part of the thyroid hormones thyroxine (T_4) and tri-iodothyronine (T_3).

Dietary sources

Fish and all seafood, seaweeds, iodised salt, milk.

Action

- An important constituent of the thyroid hormones T_4 and T_3, which are necessary for several metabolic functions, including: lipid, carbohydrate and nitrogen metabolism; growth, development and reproduction; oxygen consumption; and regulation of basal metabolic rate.
- Plays an important role in fetal brain development independent of its action via thyroid hormones.

Possible uses

Health effect or disease risk	Strength of evidence
Preventing/treating iodine deficiency, including goitre	C

C, convincing.

Bioavailability

Iodine is rapidly and almost completely absorbed and transported to the thyroid gland, where it is found in greatest concentration, although all body tissues and secretions contain trace amounts. Excretion is mainly in the urine.

Precautions/contraindications

None reported.

Pregnancy/breastfeeding

Doses exceeding the RDA should not be used (they may result in abnormal thyroid function in the infant).

Adverse effects

Hyperthyroidism, toxic modular goitre or hypothyroidism in autoimmune thyroid disease; risk of hyperkalaemia with prolonged use of high doses. Toxicity is rare with intakes < 5000 mcg daily and extremely rare at intakes < 1000 mcg daily. Hypersensitivity reactions including headache, rashes, symptoms of head cold, swelling of lips, throat and tongue, and arthralgia (joint pain) have been reported.

Interactions

Drugs

Antithyroid drugs: iodine may interfere with thyroid control.

Dose

Iodine is available mostly as an ingredient in multivitamin and mineral products. Dietary supplements usually provide 50–100% of the RDA.

Iron

Description

Iron is an essential trace mineral.

Human requirements

DRVs for iron							
Age	UK				USA		FAO/WHO
	LNRI (mg/ day)	EAR (mg/ day)	RNI (mg/ day)	EVM (mg/ day)	RDA (mg/ day)	TUL (mg/ day)	RNI[g] (mg/ day)
0–3 months	0.9	1.3	1.7		0.27[e]	40	–
4–6 months	2.3	3.3	4.3		0.27[e]	40	–
7–12 months	4.2	6.0	7.8		11	40	6.2–18.6
1–3 years	3.7	5.3	6.9		7	40	3.9–11.6
4–6 years	3.3	4.7	6.1		–	–	4.2–12.6
4–8 years	–	–	–		10	40	–
7–10 years	4.7	6.7	8.7		10	–	5.9–17.8[b]
9–13 years	–	–	–		8	40	–
Males							
11–14 years	6.1	8.7	11.3		–	–	9.7–29.2[c]
15–18 years	6.1	8.7	11.3		–	–	12.5–37.6
14–18 years	–	–	–		11	45	–
19–50+ years	4.7	6.7	8.7	17	8	45	9.2–27.4
Females							
11–14 years	8.0	11.4	14.8[d]		–	–	9.3–28.0[c,h]/ 21.8–65.4[c,i]

14–18 years	–	–	–		15	45	–
15–50+ years	8.0	11.4	14.8[d]	17	–	–	–
19–50 years	–	–	–		18	45	19.6–58.8
50+ years	4.7	6.7	8.7		8	45	9.1–27.4
Pregnancy	[a]	[a]	[a]		27	45	NS
Lactation	[a]	[a]	[a]		9[f]	45	10.0–30.0
Post–menopause						8	
Pre–menopause					18		

EU RDA = 14 mg

EAR, estimated average requirement; EU RDA, European Union recommended daily allowance; EVM, likely safe daily intake from supplements alone; LNRI, lower reference nutrient intake; RDA, recommended daily allowance; RNI, reference nutrient intake; TUL, tolerable upper intake level.

[a]No increment.

[b]7–9 years.

[c]10–14 years.

[d]Insufficient level for women who have high menstrual losses who may need iron supplements.

[e]Adequate intakes (AIs).

[f]Aged <18 years, 10 mg daily.

[g]Requirement depends on iron bioavailability of the diet.

[h]Premenarche.

[i]Postmenarche.

Dietary intake

In the UK, the average adult diet provides: for men 13.2 mg daily; for women, 10.0 mg daily. Dietary iron consists of haem and non-haem iron; in animal foods, about 40% of the iron is haem iron and 60% non-haem iron; all the iron in vegetable products is non-haem iron. Haem iron is absorbed more efficiently than non-haem iron and is independent of vitamin C. Absorption of non-haem iron can be enhanced by vitamin C (when consumed together); it can be inhibited by bran, phytates and polyphenols in tea.

Action

Iron is a component of haemoglobin, myoglobin and many enzymes involved in a variety of metabolic functions, including transport and storage of oxygen, the electron transport chain, DNA synthesis and catecholamine metabolism.

Dietary sources

Liver, red meats, egg yolk, seafood, wholegrain and enriched cereals, dried fruit.

Possible uses

Health effect or disease risk	Strength of evidence
Preventing/treating iron deficiency	C

C, convincing.

Bioavailability

Ferrous salts are more efficiently absorbed than ferric salts.

Precautions/contraindications

Conditions associated with iron overload (e.g. haemochromatosis, haemosiderosis, thalassaemia) and gastrointestinal disease, particularly inflammatory bowel disease, intestinal stricture, diverticulitis and peptic ulcer.

Pregnancy/breastfeeding

Monitor iron status. Routine iron prescription not recommended in pregnancy.

Adverse effects

Iron supplements may cause gastrointestinal irritation, nausea and constipation, which may lead to faecal impaction, particularly in elderly people. Patients with inflammatory bowel disease may suffer exacerbation of diarrhoea. Any reduced incidence of side effects associated with modified-release preparations may be caused by the fact that only small amounts of iron are released in the intestine. Liquid iron preparations may stain the teeth.

Interactions

Drugs

Antacids: reduced absorption of iron; give 2 h apart.
Bisphosphonates: reduced absorption of bisphosphonates; give 2 h apart.
Co-careldopa: reduced plasma levels of carbidopa and levodopa.
Levodopa: absorption of levodopa may be reduced.
Methyldopa: reduced absorption of methyldopa.
Penicillamine: reduced absorption of penicillamine.

4-Quinolones: absorption of ciprofloxacin, norfloxacin and ofloxacin reduced by oral iron; give 2 h apart.
Tetracyclines: reduced absorption of iron and vice versa; give 2 h apart.
Trientine: reduced absorption of iron; give 2 h apart.

Nutrients

Calcium: calcium carbonate or calcium phosphate may reduce absorption of iron; give 2 h apart (absorption of iron in multiple formulations containing iron and calcium is not significantly altered).
Copper: large doses of iron may reduce copper status and vice versa.
Manganese: reduced absorption of manganese.
Vitamin E: large doses of iron may increase requirement for vitamin E; vitamin E may impair haematological response to iron in patients with iron-deficiency anaemia.
Zinc: reduced absorption of iron and vice versa.

Dose

As a dietary supplement (mainly in multivitamin/mineral products), 10–17 mg daily; take with food to reduce gastrointestinal irritation, but food reduces absorption.

Isoflavones

Description

Isoflavones are a group of phytoestrogens, similar chemically to the oestrogens.

Constituents

Genistein, daidzein, glycetin.

Dietary sources

Soya beans and soya products (e.g. soya flour, soya milk, tempeh, tofu) are the most abundant sources containing 0.2–1.6 mg/g dry weight. Smaller amounts are found in chickpeas, flax and other seeds.

Action

Isoflavones bind to one of the subtypes of the oestrogen receptor (ERβ), whereas mammalian oestradiol has a higher binding affinity for the classic oestrogen receptor (ERα). Isoflavones can thus act as oestrogen agonists or antagonists.

Isoflavones may arrest growth of cancer cells through inhibition of DNA replication, interference of signal transduction pathways and reduction in the activity of various enzymes. They also exhibit antioxidant effects, suppress angiogenesis, and inhibit the actions of various growth factors and cytokines.

Possible uses[1–6]

Health effect or disease risk	Strength of evidence
Reduces cholesterol	
Soya protein	P
Isoflavone supplements	I

Reduces risk of breast and colorectal cancer	
Soya foods	PR
Isoflavone supplements	I
Reduces risk of osteoporosis	
Soya foods	I
Isoflavone supplements	I
Treats menopausal symptoms	
Soya foods	P
Isoflavone supplements	I
Improves cognitive function	I

I, insufficient; P, possible; PR, probable.

Bioavailability

Isoflavones are efficiently absorbed from the gastrointestinal tract with extensive tissue distribution after absorption and peak plasma concentrations.[7] Analysis of 33 isoflavone supplements found considerable differences in the isoflavone content (and therefore bioavailability) from that claimed by manufacturers.[7]

Precautions/contraindications

Hormone-dependent cancers (e.g. breast cancer).

Pregnancy/breastfeeding

No problems reported, but insufficient data. As a result of hormonal effects, isoflavones are probably best avoided.

Adverse effects

May stimulate cell proliferation in breast cancer.

Interactions

None reported.

Dose

Not established. Supplements provide 50–100 mg/dose.

References

1. Williamson-Hughes PS, Flickinger BD, Messina MJ, Empie MW. Isoflavone supplements containing predominantly genistein reduce hot flash symptoms: a critical review of published studies. *Menopause* 2006; 13: 831–839.
2. Dewell A, Hollenbeck PL, Hollenbeck CB. Clinical review: a critical evaluation of the role of soy protein and isoflavone supplementation in the control of plasma cholesterol concentrations. *J Clin Endocrinol Metab* 2006; 91: 772–780.
3. Taku K, Umegaki K, Sato Y, Taki Y, Endoh K, Watanabe S. Soy isoflavones lower serum total and LDL cholesterol in humans: a meta-analysis of 11 randomized controlled trials. *Am J Clin Nutr* 2007; 85: 1148–1156.
4. Messina M, Hughes C. Efficacy of soyfoods and soybean isoflavone supplements for alleviating menopausal symptoms is positively related to initial hot flush frequency. *J Med Food* 2003; 6: 1–11.
5. Sarkar FH, Li Y. Soy isoflavones and cancer prevention. *Cancer Invest* 2003; 21: 744–757.
6. Ishimi Y. [Prevention of osteoporosis by foods and dietary supplements. Soybean isoflavone and bone metabolism]. *Clin Calcium* 2006; 16: 1661–1667.
7. Setchell KD, Brown NM, Desai P *et al.* Bioavailability of pure isoflavones in healthy humans and analysis of commercial soy isoflavone supplements. *J Nutr* 2001; 131(suppl): S1362–S1375.

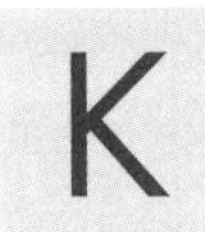

Kelp

Description

Kelp is a long-stemmed seaweed, derived from various species (e.g. *Fucus*, *Laminaria* spp.) of brown algae, known as a preparation of dried seaweed of various species.

Constituents

Iodine and other trace minerals.

Possible uses

Health effect or disease risk	Strength of evidence
Source of iodine	C
Slimming aid	I

C, convincing; I, insufficient.

Precautions/contraindications

Thyroid disorders.

Pregnancy/breastfeeding

Avoid.

Adverse effects

Hyperthyroidism or hypothyroidism. Kelp may also contain contaminants (arsenic, lead or mercury). Nausea and diarrhoea reported occasionally.

Interactions

See iodine.

Dose

Not established. Supplements contain 250–500 mg of kelp. Iodine content may not be labelled.

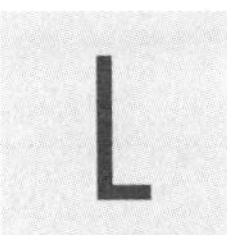

Lecithin

Description

Lecithin is a phospholipid known as phosphatidylcholine.

Constituents

Phosphatidylcholine consists of glycerol, two molecules of fatty acids, phosphoric acid and choline.

Human requirements

Lecithin is not an essential component of the diet. It is synthesised from choline.

Action

Lecithin is a source of choline when digested and a component of the lipoproteins that transport fat and cholesterol in the bloodstream. It exists within the cell as a dipolar ion; choline is a strong base and phosphoric acid is a moderately strong acid.

Dietary sources

Lecithin is a byproduct of refined soyabean oil; it is also found in eggs, red meat and nuts.

Possible uses[1,2]

Health effect or disease risk	Strength of evidence
Lowers cholesterol	I
Improvement in Alzheimer's disease	I
Improved memory and cognition	I

I, insufficient.

Bioavailability

About 50% of ingested lecithin enters the thoracic duct intact. The rest is degraded to glycerophosphorylcholine in the intestine, and then to choline in the liver. Plasma choline levels reflect lecithin intake.

Precautions/contraindications

None known.

Pregnancy/breastfeeding

No problems reported, but insufficient data for supplements.

Adverse effects

None reported.

Interactions

None reported.

Dose

Not established. Supplements provide 1200–2400 mg daily.

References

1. Higgins JPT, Flicker L. Lecithin for dementia and cognitive impairment. *Cochrane Database Syst Rev* 2000(4): CD001015.
2. Wood JL, Allison RG. Effects of consumption of choline and lecithin on neurological and cardiovascular systems. *Fed Proc* 1982; 41: 3015–3021.

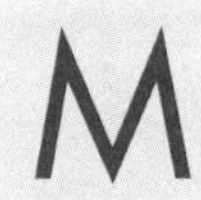

Magnesium

Description

Magnesium is an essential mineral. It is the second most abundant intracellular cation in the body.

Human requirements

DRVs for magnesium							
Age	UK				USA		WHO
	LNRI (mg/day)	EAR (mg/day)	RNI (mg/day)	EVM (mg/day)	RDA (mg/day)	TUL (mg/day)	RNI (mg/day)
0–3 months	30	40	55		30	–	26–36
4–6 months	40	50	60		30	–	26–36
7–9 months	45	60	75		75	–	54
10–12 months	45	60	80		75	–	54
1–3 years	50	65	85		80	65	60
4–6 years	70	90	120		–	–	76
4–8 years	–	–	–		130	110	–
7–10 years	115	150	200		170	–	100[b]
9–13 years	–	–	–	–	240	350	–

continued

(continued)

Males							
11–14 years	180	230	280		–	–	230[c]
14–18 years	–	–	–		410	350	230
15–18 years	190	250	280		–	–	–
19–50+ years	190	250	300	300	–	–	260[d]
19–30 years	–	–	–		400	350	–
31–70+ years	–	–	–		420	350	–
Females							
11–14 years	180	230	280		–	–	220[c]
14–18 years	–	–	–		360	350	220
15–18 years	190	250	300		310	–	–
19–50 years	190	250	300	300	280	–	260[e]
50+ years	150	200	270	300	280	–	–
19–30 years	–	–	–		310	350	–
31–70+ years	–	–	–		320	350	–
Pregnancy	[a]	[a]	[a]	360–400	350	220	
Lactation			+50		320–360	350	270

EU RDA = 14 mg.
EAR, estimated average requirement; EU RDA, European Union recommended daily allowance; EVM, likely safe daily intake from supplements alone; LNRI, lower reference nutrient intake; RDA, recommended daily allowance; RNI, reference nutrient intake; TUL, tolerable upper intake level.
[a] No increment.
[b] 7–9 years.
[c] 10–14 years.
[d] >65 years = 224 mg.
[e] >65 years = 190 mg.

Dietary intake

In the UK, the average diet provides: for males, 336 mg daily; for females, 250 mg daily.

Action

- An essential cofactor for enzymes requiring ATP (these are involved in glycolysis, fatty acid oxidation and amino acid metabolism).
- Required for the synthesis of RNA and replication of DNA.
- Plays a role in neuromuscular transmission and calcium metabolism.
- Inhibits vascular smooth muscle contraction.
- Helps to regulate blood pressure.

Dietary sources

Legumes, nuts, unrefined grains, cocoa, soya beans, dark-green leafy vegetables, seafood.

Possible uses[1–6]

Health effect or disease risk	Strength of evidence
Protects against coronary heart disease (CHD)	P
Improves outcomes in CHD	P
Lowers blood pressure	P
Improves metabolic control in patients with diabetes mellitus who are low in magnesium	P
Improves premenstrual syndrome	P
Alleviates migraine headaches	I
Improves bone density in older people	P
Improves athletic performance	I

I, insufficient; P, possible.

Bioavailability

Magnesium is readily absorbed and distributed in the skeleton and soft tissues. Magnesium citrate is more soluble and bioavailable than magnesium oxide.

Precautions/contraindications

Doses exceeding the RDA should be avoided in renal impairment.

Pregnancy/breastfeeding

No problems reported with normal intakes.

Adverse effects

Toxicity unlikely if renal function normal. Doses of 3–5 g may be cathartic.

Interactions

Drugs

Alcohol: excessive alcohol intake increases renal excretion of magnesium.
Loop diuretics: increased excretion of magnesium.
4-Quinolones: may reduce absorption of 4-quinolones; give 2 h apart.
Tetracyclines: may reduce absorption of tetracyclines; give 2 h apart.
Thiazide diuretics: increased excretion of magnesium.

Dose

Not established. Dietary supplements provide 100–500 mg/dose.

References

1. Ueshima K. Magnesium and ischemic heart disease: a review of epidemiological, experimental, and clinical evidences. *Magnes Res* 2005; 18: 275–284.
2. Belin RJ, He K. Magnesium physiology and pathogenic mechanisms that contribute to the development of the metabolic syndrome. *Magnes Res* 2007; 20: 107–129.
3. He K, Song Y, Belin RJ, Chen Y. Magnesium intake and the metabolic syndrome: epidemiologic evidence to date. *J Cardiometab Syndr* 2006; 1: 351–355.
4. Barbagallo M, Dominguez LJ, Resnick LM. Magnesium metabolism in hypertension and type 2 diabetes mellitus. *Am J Ther* 2007; 14: 375–385.
5. Dickinson HO, Nicolson DJ, Campbell F *et al.* Magnesium supplementation for the management of essential hypertension in adults. *Cochrane Database Syst Rev* 2006(3): CD004640.
6. Nielsen FH, Lukaski HC. Update on the relationship between magnesium and exercise. *Magnes Res* 2006; 19: 180–189.

Manganese

Description

Manganese is an essential trace mineral. The human body contains 12–20 mg of manganese, which is concentrated in tissues rich in mitochondria, such as the pancreas, kidneys, skin and muscle.

Human requirements

DRVs for manganese				
Age	UK		USA	
	Safe intake (mg/day)	EVM (mg/day)	AI (mg/day)	TUL (mg/day)
Males and females				
0–6 months	0.01		0.003	–
7–12 months			0.6	–
1–3 years			1.2	2
4–6 years			–	–
4–8 years			1.5	3
7–9 years			–	–
9–13 years			1.9[a]/1.6[b]	6
10–18 years			–	–
14–18 years			2.2[a]/1.6[b]	9
19–50 years			2.3[a]/1.8[b]	11
51+ years			2.3[a]/1.8[b]	11
11–50+ years	1.4	4	–	–
Pregnancy			2.0	–
Lactation			2.6	

AI, adequate intake; EVM, likely safe daily intake from supplements alone; TUL, tolerable upper intake level.
[a]Males.
[b]Females.

Dietary intake

In the UK, the average adult diet provides 4.6–5.4 mg daily

Action

- Activates several enzymes, including hydroxylases, kinases, decarboxylases and transferases.
- A constituent of several metalloenzymes, such as arginase and pyruvate carboxylase, and also superoxide dismutase, which protects cells from free radical attack.
- Involved in glucose and fatty acid metabolism and urea formation.
- Needed for bone development, growth and reproduction, skin integrity and utilisation of thiamine.

Dietary sources

Nuts, legumes, unrefined grains, cocoa, coffee, tea, leafy vegetables, fruits.

Possible uses

Health effect or disease risk	Strength of evidence
Protects against oxidative damage	P
Reduces inflammation in rheumatoid arthritis	I
Improves insulin sensitivity in diabetes	I

I, insufficient; P, possible.

Precautions/contraindications

None (at normal doses).

Pregnancy/breastfeeding

No problems reported at normal doses.

Adverse effects

None at normal doses. Toxicity has occurred from drinking well water contaminated with manganese from buried batteries and prolonged exposure and inhalation of ore dust.

Interactions

None reported.

Dose

Not established. Dietary supplements provide 5–50 mg/dose.

Melatonin

Description

Melatonin, the main hormone of the pineal gland, is synthesised from the amino acid tryptophan via serotonin. Synthesis decreases with age.

Action

- Regulates sleep.
- Scavenges free radicals.
- Modulates the immune system.
- May inhibit cancer growth.

Possible uses[1–8]

Health effect or disease risk	Strength of evidence
Prevents jet lag	PR
Improved sleep latency	P
Improves insomnia in older people	P
Sleep enhancement in healthy adults	P
Sleep enhancement in Alzheimer's disease	I
Sleep enhancement in neuropsychiatric disorders	I
Attention deficit hyperactivity disorder	I
Bipolar disorder	I
Seasonal affective disorder	I
Treatment of cancer	I
Hypertension	I
Parkinson's disease	I
Chronic fatigue syndrome	I

Tardive dyskinesia	I
Irritable bowel syndrome	I
Headache prevention	I
Reduced damage post stroke	I
Osteoporosis	I
Management of glaucoma	I
Age-related macular degeneration	I[9]

I, insufficient; P, possible; PR, probable.

Bioavailability

Melatonin is rapidly absorbed and has a half-life of 45 minutes.

Precautions/contraindications

Caution in women wishing to conceive (may inhibit ovulation).

Pregnancy/breastfeeding

Avoid.

Adverse effects

No known toxicity or serious side effects, but the effects of long-term supplementation are unknown. Reports of headaches, abdominal cramp, inhibition of fertility and libido, gynaecomastia and exacerbation of symptoms of fibromyalgia, and also of sleep disturbance and increased seizures in children suffering from neurological disorders. Inhibition of ovulation has been observed with high doses, but melatonin should not be used as a contraceptive.

Interactions

No data are available, but in theory melatonin may be additive with medication that causes CNS depression. In addition, β blockers inhibit melatonin release, and this may be the mechanism by which β blockers cause sleep disturbance. Other drugs, including fluoxetine, ibuprofen and indometacin, may also reduce nocturnal melatonin secretion. Melatonin may influence the effects of warfarin.

Dose

Not established. Manufacturers recommend 3–5 mg a couple of hours before sleep time.

For jet lag, if flying eastward, take a dose at 6–7 p.m. on the day of departure then at bedtime on arrival for 2–3 days.

If flying westward (only of value if crossing four to five time zones), take a dose at bedtime on arrival; repeat for 2–3 days.

References

1. Altun A, Ugur-Altun B. Melatonin: therapeutic and clinical utilization. *Int J Clin Pract* 2007; 61: 835–845.
2. Bondy SC, Sharman EH. Melatonin and the aging brain. *Neurochem Int* 2007; 50: 571–580.
3. Jung B, Ahmad N. Melatonin in cancer management: progress and promise. *Cancer Res* 2006; 66: 9789–9793.
4. Srinivasan V, Smits M, Spence W *et al*. Melatonin in mood disorders. *World J Biol Psychiatry* 2006; 7: 138–151.
5. Vogler B, Rapoport AM, Tepper SJ, Sheftell F, Bigal ME. Role of melatonin in the pathophysiology of migraine: implications for treatment. *CNS Drugs* 2006; 20: 343–350.
6. Schernhammer E, Chen H, Ritz B. Circulating melatonin levels: possible link between Parkinson's disease and cancer risk? *Cancer Causes Control* 2006; 17: 577–582.
7. Pandi-Perumal SR, Zisapel N, Srinivasan V, Cardinali DP. Melatonin and sleep in aging population. *Exp Gerontol* 2005; 40: 911–925.
8. Herxheimer A, Petrie KJ. Melatonin for the prevention and treatment of jet lag. *Cochrane Database Syst Rev* 2002(2): D001520.
9. Lundmark PO, Pandi-Perumal SR, Srinivasan V, Cardinali DP. Role of melatonin in the eye and ocular dysfunctions. *Vis Neurosci* 2006; 23: 853–862.

Methylsulfonylmethane

Description

Methylsulfonylmethane (MSM) is an organic sulphur-containing compound. It is an oxidation product of the organic solvent, dimethylsulphoxide (DMSO).

Dietary sources

Fruits, vegetables, milk, meat, fish, coffee, tea and chocolate.

Action

Claimed to be important as a source of sulphur, but there is no evidence to support this need in humans. Sulphur can be obtained from dietary amino acids such as cysteine and methionine. Sulphur is needed for the formation of connective tissue. MSM is claimed to be a source of sulphur for building connective tissue.

Possible uses[1]

Health effect or disease risk	Strength of evidence
Pain in osteoarthritis	I
Allergic rhinitis	I
Lowers homocysteine	I

I, insufficient.

Precautions/contraindications

None reported.

Pregnancy/breastfeeding

No problems have been reported, but there have not been sufficient studies to guarantee the safety of MSM in pregnancy/breastfeeding.

Adverse effects

MSM is a component of foods and has not been reported to be toxic. No adverse effects were reported when rats were given 1–5 g/kg body weight for 3 months.[2] A 30-day study in humans revealed no side effects with a 2600 mg daily dosage.[3]

Interactions

None reported.

Dose

The dose is not established. Supplements typically provide 1500–3000 mg in a daily dose.

References

1. Monograph. Methylsulfonylmethane (MSM). *Altern Med Rev* 2003; 8: 438–441.

2. Horvath K, Noker PE, Somfai-Relle S, *et al.* Toxicity of methylsulfonylmethane in rats. *Food Chem Toxicol* 2002; 40: 1459–1462.

3. Barrager E, Veltmann JR. Jr, Schauss AG, Schiller RN. A multicentered, open-label trial on the safety and efficacy of methylsulfonylmethane in the treatment of seasonal allergic rhinitis. *J Altern Complement Med* 2002; 8: 167–173.

Molybdenum

Description

Molybdenum is an essential ultratrace mineral.

Human requirements

DRVs for molybdenum			
Age	UK	USA	
	Safe intake (mcg/kg/day)	AI (mcg/day)	TUL (mcg/day)
Males and females			
0–6 months	0.5–1.5	2	
7–12 months	0.5–1.5	3	
1–3 years	0.5–1.5	17	300
4–8 years	0.5–1.5	22	600
9–13 years	0.5–1.5	34	1100
14–18 years	0.5–1.5	43	1700
19–70+ years	50–400 mcg/day	45	2000
Pregnancy	50–400 mcg/day	50	1700
Lactation	50–400 mcg/day	50	2000

AI, adequate intake; TUL, tolerable upper intake level.

Dietary intake

Average adult intakes of molybdenum are 120–140 mcg daily (US figures).

Action

A constituent of three enzymes involved in the metabolism of sulphur and purines and the transfer of electrons for the oxidation/reduction process.

Dietary sources

Organ meats (e.g. offal), milk and milk products, whole grains, legumes, cereals and dark-green leafy vegetables.

Possible uses

None established.

Precautions/contraindications

None in usual doses.

Pregnancy/breastfeeding

No problems in usual dosage.

Adverse effects

Molybdenum is a relatively non-toxic element. High dietary intakes (10–15 mg daily) have been associated with elevated uric acid concentrations in blood, an increased incidence of gout and altered metabolism of nucleotides.

Interactions

High doses may impair bioavailability of copper.

Dose

Molybdenum is available mainly in multivitamin and mineral supplements. There is no established dose.

Multivitamins

Description

Multivitamins are dietary supplements containing a variety of vitamins and minerals.[1] There are three main categories:

1 Products containing 10 or more vitamins and minerals, often in amounts around the recommended daily amount (RDA).
2 Products containing vitamins and minerals in higher than RDA doses (may be labelled high potency).
3 Products containing a few vitamins and minerals (e.g. up to six) which may be marketed for special life stages and purposes (e.g. menopause, sports, pregnancy, children, vegetarians).

Action

Specific potential benefits depend on vitamins and minerals in the product. Vitamins and minerals are important for good health: normal growth and development, overall health and well-being, release of energy from food, healthy teeth and bones, healing and repair of body tissue, healthy eyes, normal healthy structure of skin, hair and nails, and the health of muscles, the nervous system and the circulatory system.

Possible uses[2–12]

Health effect or disease risk	Strength of evidence
Protect against dietary gaps of vitamins and minerals	C
Reduce proportions of individuals who do not achieve recommended intakes	C
Improve vitamin and mineral intakes	C
Improve plasma levels of vitamins and minerals	C
Reduce proportions of individuals with suboptimal intakes	C
Reduced risk of cancer	I

continued

(continued)

Reduce risk of cardiovascular disease	I
Improved cognitive function	I
Reduce risk of infection	I
Reduce risk of cataract	I
Reduce risk of macular degeneration	I

C, convincing; I, insufficient.

Precautions

Care should be taken not to exceed safe upper levels of any vitamin and mineral, particularly if taken long term. Caution should be exercised if multivitamins are taken with one or several other dietary supplements.

Adverse effects[13]

Multivitamin products containing the RDA of vitamins and minerals are generally thought to be safe.

Interactions

- Multivitamins may affect warfarin anticoagulation in susceptible patients.
- See also monographs on individual vitamins and minerals.

References

1. Yetley EA. Multivitamin and multimineral dietary supplements: definitions, characterization, bioavailability, and drug interactions. *Am J Clin Nutr* 2007; 85: S269–S276.
2. Troppmann L, Gray-Donald K, Johns T. Supplement use: is there any nutritional benefit? *J Am Diet Assoc* 2002; 102: 818–825.
3. Sebastian RS, Cleveland LE, Goldman JD, Moshfegh AJ. Older adults who use vitamin/mineral supplements differ from nonusers in nutrient intake adequacy and dietary attitudes. *J Am Diet Assoc* 2007; 107: 1322–1332.
4. Stephen AI, Avenell A. A systematic review of multivitamin and multimineral supplementation for infection. *J Hum Nutr Diet* 2006; 19: 179–190.
5. Murphy SP, White KK, Park SY, Sharma S. Multivitamin-multimineral supplements' effect on total nutrient intake. *Am J Clin Nutr* 2007; 85: S280–S284.
6. Mason P. One is okay, more is better? Pharmacological aspects and safe limits of nutritional supplements. *Proc Nutr Soc* 2007; 66: 493–507.
7. Liu BA, McGeer A, McArthur MA *et al.* Effect of multivitamin and mineral supplementation on episodes of infection in nursing home residents: a randomized, placebo-controlled study. *J Am Geriatr Soc* 2007; 55: 35–42.

8. Huang HY, Caballero B, Chang S *et al*. Multivitamin/mineral supplements and prevention of chronic disease. *Evid Rep Technol Assess (Full Rep)* 2006 (139): 1–117.

9. Huang HY, Caballero B, Chang S *et al*. The efficacy and safety of multivitamin and mineral supplement use to prevent cancer and chronic disease in adults: a systematic review for a National Institutes of Health state-of-the-science conference. *Ann Intern Med* 2006; 145: 372–385.

10. Greenwald P, Anderson D, Nelson SA, Taylor PR. Clinical trials of vitamin and mineral supplements for cancer prevention. *Am J Clin Nutr* 2007; 85: S314–S317.

11. Avenell A, Campbell MK, Cook JA *et al*. Effect of multivitamin and multimineral supplements on morbidity from infections in older people (MAVIS trial): pragmatic, randomised, double blind, placebo controlled trial. *BMJ* 2005; 331: 324–329.

12. El-Kadiki A, Sutton AJ. Role of multivitamins and mineral supplements in preventing infections in elderly people: systematic review and meta-analysis of randomised controlled trials. *BMJ* 2005; 330: 871.

13. Mulholland CA, Benford DJ. What is known about the safety of multivitamin-multimineral supplements for the generally healthy population? Theoretical basis for harm. *Am J Clin Nutr* 2007; 85: S318–S322.

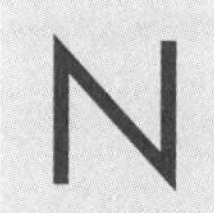

N-Acetylcysteine

Description

N-Acetylcysteine (NAC) is the acetylated form of the amino acid cysteine found naturally in foods.

Action

- NAC is the precursor of glutathione, which functions as a detoxicant and antioxidant in the body.
- Chelates heavy metals such as cadmium.

Possible uses

Health effect or disease risk	Strength of evidence
Chronic bronchitis	P
COPD	I
Prevention of influenza	P
Supplementation of anti-retroviral therapy in HIV/AIDS	P
Prevention of lung cancer	I

I, insufficient; P, possible.
COPD, chronic obstructive pulmonary disease.

Precautions/contraindications

None reported.

Pregnancy/breastfeeding

No problems reported, but insufficient data.

Adverse effects

None reported.

Interactions

None reported.

Dose

Not established. Clinical trials have used 600–1200 mg daily.

Niacin

Description

Niacin is a water-soluble vitamin of the vitamin B complex. Niacin is a generic term used to describe the compounds that exhibit the biological properties of nicotinamide. It occurs in food as nicotinamide and nicotinic acid. It is sometimes known as niacinamide.

Human requirements

DRVs for niacin (nicotinic acid equivalent)								
Age	UK					USA		FAO/ WHO
	LNRI (mg/ 1000 kcal)[a]	EAR (mg/ 1000 kcal)	RNI (mg/ 1000 kcal)	RNI (mg/ day)	EVM (mg/ day)	RDA (mg/ day)	TUL (mg/ day)	RNI (mg/ day)
0–6 months	4.4	5.5	6.6	3		2	–	2
7–12 months	4.4	5.5	6.6	5		3	–	4
1–3 years	4.4	5.5	6.6	8		6	10	6
4–6 years	4.4	5.5	6.6	11		–	–	9
4–8 years		–	–	–		8	15	–
7–10 years	4.4	5.5	6.6	12		–	–	12[b]
9–13 years	–	–	–	–		12	20	–
Males								
11–14 years	4.4	5.5	6.6	15		–	–	16[c]
15–18 years	4.4	5.5	6.6	18		–	–	16
14–18 years	–	–	–	–		16	30	–
19–50 years	4.4	5.5	6.6	17	17[d]	16	35	16

continued

(continued)

51–65+ years	–	–	–	–		–	–	16
51–70+ years	–	–	–	–		16	35	–
Females								
11–14ye ars	4.4	5.5	6.6	12		–	–	14[c]
15–18 years	4.4	5.5	6.6	14		–	–	14
14–18 years	–	–	–	–		14	30	–
19–50 years	4.4	5.5	6.6	13	17[d]	14	35	14
51–65+ years	–	–	–	–		–	–	14
51–70+ years	–	–	–	–		14	35	–
Pregnancy	a	a	a	–		18	35[e]	18
Lactation	a	a	+2.3	+2		17	35[e]	17

EU RDA = 18 mg.

EAR, estimated average requirement; EU RDA, European Union recommended daily allowance; EVM, likely safe daily intake from supplements alone; LNRI, lower reference nutrient intake; RDA, recommended daily allowance; RNI, reference nutrient intake; TUL, tolerable upper intake level.

[a]No increment.

[b]7–9 years.

[c]10–14 years.

[d]Likely safe daily intake of nicotinamide from supplements alone is 500 mg daily.

[e]Women <18 years = 30 mg daily.

Dietary intake

In the UK, the average adult diet provides (niacin equivalents): for men, 44.7 mg daily; for women, 30.9 mg daily.

Action

Nicotinamide is a constituent of two coenzymes: nicotinamide adenine dinucleotide (NAD) and nicotinamide adenine dinucleotide phosphate (NADP), which act as hydrogen and electron acceptors and donors, respectively; they function in the metabolism of carbohydrate, fat and protein, rhodopsin synthesis and cellular respiration.

Nicotinic acid in pharmacological doses is a peripheral vasodilator; it reduces LDL-cholesterol, raises HDL-cholesterol and lowers triglycerides.

Dietary sources

Niacin is found in most animal and plant foods but often in a form that is unavailable. Good sources are meats, fish, poultry, liver, eggs, milk, legumes, nuts and enriched cereals. Another source is biosynthesis from the amino acid, tryptophan (1 mg niacin ≡ 60 mg tryptophan).

Possible uses[1]

Health effect or disease risk	Strength of evidence
Lowers cholesterol (nicotinic acid in pharmacological doses)	C

C, convincing.

Bioavailability

Lack of sufficient data.

Precautions/contraindications

Gout, peptic ulcer and liver disease. High doses should be avoided in diabetes.

Pregnancy/breastfeeding

No problems reported.

Adverse effects

Nicotinamide (doses >3 g/day for 3 months): nausea, headaches, heartburn, fatigue, sore throat, dry hair, dry skin and blurred vision.
Nicotinic acid: skin flushing, severe itching, gastrointestinal disturbances; long-term use may cause xerostomia, activation of peptic ulcer, blurred vision, hyperglycaemia, jaundice and liver damage.

Interactions

Drugs

Lipid-lowering drugs: increased risk of rhabdomyolysis and myopathy (combined therapy should include careful monitoring).

Nutrients

Adequate amounts of all B vitamins are required for optimal functioning; deficiency or excess of one B vitamin may lead to abnormalities in the metabolism of another.

Dose

Nicotinamide is available in the form of tablets, but is found mainly in multivitamin and mineral products.

Dietary supplements generally provide 30–50 mg daily.

Reference

1. Carlson LA. Nicotinic acid: the broad-spectrum lipid drug. A 50th anniversary review. *J Intern Med* 2005; 258: 94–114.

Nickel

Description

A trace element essential to several animals. Essentiality in humans is unproven.

Human requirements

Not established. The US Food and Nutrition Board set a tolerable upper intake level (TUL) of 1 mg daily for adolescents and all adults.

Dietary intake

Mean intake of dietary nickel in the UK is 130 mcg daily, with an estimated maximum intake of 260 mcg daily.

Action

Present in DNA and RNA; a cofactor or structural component in specific enzymes involved in intermediary metabolism.

Dietary sources

Nickel is present in a variety of foods, particularly pulses, grains (especially oats) and nuts. It is also present in drinking water.

Possible uses

None established.

Bioavailability

Lack of sufficient data.

Precautions/contraindications

None reported.

Pregnancy/breastfeeding

No problems reported at usual exposure from food.

Adverse effects

None reported at usual exposure from food. Chronic exposure in animals is associated with degeneration of heart muscle, brain, lung, liver and kidney. A cause of allergic contact dermatitis.

Interactions

Nickel interacts with most minerals, especially it enhances absorption and metabolism of iron.

Drugs

None reported.

Dose

Not established.

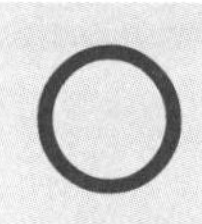

Octacosanol

Description

Octacosanol is the main component of policosanol, which is isolated from sugar cane wax, *Eupolyphaga sinensis*, some *Euphorbia* species, *Acacia modeseta, Serenoa repens* and other plants, including wholegrains, fruit and vegetables. It is a 28-carbon long-chain alcohol.

Action

Claimed to have a lipid-lowering effect.

Possible uses

Health effect or disease risk	Strength of evidence
Lowers serum cholesterol	a
Reduces platelet aggregation	I
Improves intermittent claudication	I
Improve symptoms of amyotrophic lateral sclerosis	I
Improves symptoms of Parkinson's disease	I

[a]Evidence that octacosonal lowers serum cholesterol is powerful from more than 30 randomised controlled trials (RCTs), but these have all been conducted by one research group in Cuba. Trials conducted outside of Cuba have not shown positive effects.
I, insufficient.

Bioavailability

Lack of sufficient data.

Precautions/contraindications

None reported.

Pregnancy/breastfeeding

No problems reported, but no study data in pregnant women.

Adverse effects

None reported.

Interactions

None reported.

Dose

Not established. Doses used in studies are 1–20 mg policosanol daily.

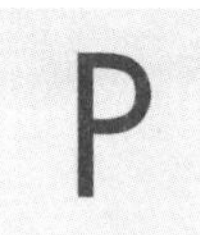

Pangamic acid

Description

A natural substance: D-gluconodimethyl aminoacetic acid (vitamin B_{15}).

Human requirements

No evidence of a requirement for pangamic acid despite its alternative name vitamin B_{15}.

Action

Little is known about the role of pangamic acid, although enhanced oxygen uptake and better adaptation to hypoxia and strenuous exercise had been reported by scientists in the former Soviet Union.

Dietary sources

Pangamic acid is a natural substance, present in foods, that was first prepared from apricot pits, and later from rice, liver, blood and yeast.

Possible uses

Pangamic acid is claimed to enhance athletic performance and to be beneficial in cardiovascular disease (CVD), asthma and diabetes mellitus. Scientific studies show no evidence of therapeutic efficacy for pangamic acid.

Precautions/contraindications

Pangamic acid should be avoided.

Pregnancy/breastfeeding

Pangamic acid should be avoided.

Adverse effects

Possibly mutagenic (causing cancer); causes transient skin flushing.

Interactions

None.

Dose

Not to be taken.

Pantothenic acid

Description

Pantothenic acid is a water-soluble B complex vitamin (derived from the Greek word meaning 'from everywhere').

Human requirements

DRVs for pantothenic acid					
Age	UK		USA		FAO/WHO
	Safe intake (mg/day)	EVM (mg/day)	AI (mg/day)	TUL (mg/day)	RNI (mg/day)
0–6 months	1.7		1.7	–	1.7
7–12 months	1.7		1.8	–	1.8
1–3 years	1.7		2.0	–	2.0
4–10 years	3–7		–	–	3.0,[a] 4.0[b]
4–8 years				3.0	
9–13 years			4.0	–	
Males and females					
11–50+ years	3–7	200	–	5.0	
14–70+ years			5.0	–	–
Pregnancy	–		6.0	–	6.0
Lactation	–		7.0	–	7.0

EU RDA = 6 mg.

AI, adequate intake; EU RDA, European Union recommended daily allowance; EVM, likely safe daily intake from supplements alone; RNI, reference nutrient intake; TUL, tolerable upper intake level.

[a]4–6 years.

[b]7–9 years.

Dietary intake

In the UK, the average adult diet provides 5.1 mg daily.

Action

Pantothenic acid is a component of coenzyme A, which functions in the metabolism of carbohydrate, protein and fat. It is also necessary for the maintenance of normal skin and for the development of the central nervous system.

Dietary sources

Widely distributed in foods. Good sources are liver, egg, meat, wholegrain cereals and legumes.

Possible uses

Pantothenic acid has been claimed to be useful in wide variety of conditions (e.g. acne, alopecia, allergies, burning feet, asthma, grey hair, dandruff, cholesterol lowering, improving exercise performance, depression, osteoarthritis, rheumatoid arthritis, multiple sclerosis, stress, shingles, ageing and Parkinson's disease). However, there is insufficient evidence for these claims.

Precautions/contraindications

None

Pregnancy/breastfeeding

No problems reported.

Adverse effects

Large amounts may cause diarrhoea and water retention.

Interactions

Drugs

Alcohol: excessive alcohol intake may increase requirement for pantothenic acid.
Oral contraceptives: may increase requirement for pantothenic acid.

Nutrients

Adequate amounts of all B vitamins are required for optimal functioning; deficiency or excess of one B vitamin may lead to abnormalities in the metabolism of another.

Dose

Not established (other than DRVs).

Para-amino benzoic acid

Description

Para-amino benzoic acid (PABA) is a member of the vitamin B complex, but is not an officially recognised vitamin.

Human requirements

None.

Action

Plays an indirect role as a component of folic acid.

Dietary sources

Brewers' yeast, kidney, liver, molasses, wheatgerm, bran and wholegrains.

Possible uses

PABA is claimed to prevent greying hair and to be useful as an anti-ageing supplement. It has been used in digestive disorders, arthritis, insomnia and depression. There is no convincing scientific evidence available.

Precautions/contraindications

None reported.

Pregnancy/breastfeeding

No problems reported, but supplements best avoided.

Adverse effects

Toxicity is low, but high doses (>30 mg) may cause anorexia, nausea, vomiting, liver toxicity, fever, itching and skin rash.

Interactions

Drugs

Sulphonamides: kill bacteria by mimicking PABA; supplements containing PABA should be avoided while taking these drugs.

Dose

No established dose. Supplements are not justified. Dietary supplements provide 100–500 mg/dose.

Pycnogenol

Description

Pycnogenol is a registered tradename for a specific standardised extract of procyanidins (a category of flavonoids) from the bark of the French maritime pine (*Pinus pinaster* ssp. *atlantica*), which is grown in the Bay of Biscay in south-west France.

Action

Stimulates production of nitric oxide and has a wide variety of effects including:

- Inhibition of platelet aggregation and improved vasodilatation.
- Inhibition of angiotensin-converting enzyme (ACE).
- Improved endothelial function.
- Improved lipid profiles.
- Enhanced capillary integrity and stabilisation of cell membranes.
- Improved erectile function.
- Antioxidant activity.
- Enhanced immune function.

Possible uses[1]

Health effect or disease risk	Strength of evidence
Reduces blood pressure	I
Reduces cardiovascular disease	I
Reduces chronic venous insufficiency	P
Prevention of deep vein thrombosis	I
Analgesic	I
Improves diabetic control	I
Alleviates attention deficit hyperactivity disorder (ADHD) in children	I

I, insufficient; P, possible.

Precautions/contraindications

None reported.

Pregnancy/breastfeeding

No teratogenic effects have been observed, but pycnogenol should be avoided as a general precaution.

Adverse effects

No serious side effects reported. Mild side effects, such as gastrointestinal problems, nausea, headache, dizziness and skin sensitisation, are rare and transient in most cases.

Interactions

None reported.

Dose

The dose is not established. Clinical trials have used 40–100 mg pycnogenol daily or 1 mg/kg body weight daily.

Reference

1. Rohdewald P. A review of the French maritime pine bark extract (Pycnogenol), a herbal medication with a diverse clinical pharmacology. *Int J Clin Pharmacol Ther* 2002; 40: 158–168.

Phosphatidylserine

Description

Phosphatidylserine is a natural component of the brain cortex and the major phospholipid in the outer surface of the brain's synaptic membranes.

Action

Plays an important role in signal transduction, secretory vesicle release and cell-to-cell communication.

Possible uses

Health effect or disease risk	Strength of evidence
Improves attention, mood and memory in Alzheimer's disease	P
Improves attention, mood and memory in Parkinson's disease	P
Improvements in depressive disorders	P
Improves physical stress response	P
Improves psychological stress response	P

P, possible.

Precautions/contraindications

None reported (except concerns about supplements made from bovine tissue because of risk of bovine spongiform encephalopathy).

Pregnancy/breastfeeding

No problems reported, but insufficient study data.

Adverse effects

None reported.

Interactions

None reported.

Dose

Not established; doses of 300–1000 mg daily used in studies.

Phytosterols

Description

Phytosterols are plant sterols with a similar structure to cholesterol. Some are unsaturated with a double bond in the chemical structure (e.g. β-sitosterol, campesterol and stigmasterol), whereas others are saturated with no double bond (e.g. sitostanol and campestanol). Phytosterols stabilise the phospholipid bilayers in plant cell membranes, as cholesterol does in animal cell membranes.

Dietary intake

Daily intake from the diet is 100–400 mg.

Action

Phyosterols reduce total cholesterol and LDL-cholesterol in blood, mainly by reducing absorption of cholesterol.

Dietary sources

All plant foods. Nuts, seeds and grains are the most concentrated sources.

Possible uses[a1–4]

Health effect or disease risk	Strength of evidence
Reduce cholesterol and LDL-cholesterol	C
Reduce cardiovascular risk	I
Reduce cancer risk	I

[a]Most evidence derived from studies with phytosterols added to foods (e.g. spreads); preliminary evidence also from food supplements.
C, convincing; I, insufficient.

Bioavailability

Absorption of phytosterols is 2–5%.

Precautions/contraindications

Avoid in phytosterolaemia (a rare genetic disorder) or in people heterozygous for the disorder. Avoid in children aged under 5 years.

Pregnancy/breastfeeding

No data in pregnant and breastfeeding women.

Adverse effects

None known.

Interactions

Drugs

Statins: possible additive effect in cholesterol lowering with phytosterols.

Nutrients

Fat-soluble vitamins: possibly reduced absorption of fat-soluble vitamins with phytosterols but evidence conflicting.

Dose

Doses used in clinical studies with phytosterol incorporated in spreads are 1–3 g daily phytosterol equivalent.

References

1. Ostlund RE, Jr. Phytosterols, cholesterol absorption and healthy diets. *Lipids* 2007; 42: 41–45.
2. Earnest CP, Mikus CR, Lemieux I, Arsenault BJ, Church TS. Examination of encapsulated phytosterol ester supplementation on lipid indices associated with cardiovascular disease. *Nutrition* 2007; 23: 625–633.
3. Woodgate D, Chan CH, Conquer JA. Cholesterol-lowering ability of a phytostanol softgel supplement in adults with mild to moderate hypercholesterolemia. *Lipids* 2006; 41: 127–132.
4. Acuff RV, Cai DJ, Dong ZP, Bell D. The lipid lowering effect of plant sterol ester capsules in hypercholesterolemic subjects. *Lipids Health Dis* 2007; 6: 11.

Potassium

Description

Potassium is an essential mineral.

Human requirements

DRVs for potassium			
Age	LRNI (mg/day)	RNI[b] (mg/day)	US minimum requirement
0–3 months	400	800	500
4–6 months	400	850	500
7–9 months	400	700	700
10–12 months	450	700	700
1–3 years	450	800	1000
4–6 years	600	1100	1400
7–10 years	950	2200	1600
11–14 years	1600	3100	2000
15–50+ years	2000	3500	2000
Pregnancy	a	a	a
Lactation	a	a	a

EU RDA = none.

EAR, estimated average requirement; EU RDA, European Union recommended daily allowance; LNRI, lower reference nutrient intake; RNI, reference nutrient intake.

[a]No increment.

[b]Desirable intakes may exceed these values.

Note: no EAR has been derived for potassium.

Dietary intake

In the UK, the average adult diet provides: for men 3279 mg daily; for women 2562 mg.

Action

Potassium is the principal intracellular cation and is fundamental to the regulation of acid–base and water balance. It contributes to transmission of nerve impulses, control of skeletal muscle contractility and maintenance of blood pressure.

Dietary sources

Bran cereals, muesli, potatoes, fish, meat, lentils, baked beans, chickpeas, bananas, dates, figs and cantaloupe melons.

Possible uses

Health effect or disease risk	Strength of evidence
Reduces blood pressure	I

I, insufficient.

Precautions

Avoid in patients with chronic renal failure (particularly in elderly people), gastrointestinal obstruction or ulceration, peptic ulcer, Addison's disease, heart block, severe burns or acute dehydration.

Pregnancy/breastfeeding

No data are available on potassium supplements in pregnancy. They should be avoided.

Adverse effects

Nausea, vomiting, diarrhoea and abdominal cramps may occur, particularly if potassium is taken on an empty stomach. Modified-release preparations may cause gastrointestinal ulceration. Hyperkalaemia is almost unknown with oral administration provided that renal function is normal. Intakes exceeding 17 g daily (unlikely from oral supplements) would be required to cause toxicity.

Interactions

Drugs

ACE inhibitors: increased risk of hyperkalaemia.
Carbenoxolone: reduced serum potassium levels.
Corticosteroids: increased excretion of potassium.
Ciclosporin: increased risk of hyperkalaemia.
Laxatives: chronic use reduces absorption of potassium.
Loop diuretics: increased risk of hypokalaemia (but potassium supplements seldom necessary with small dose of diuretic).
Non-steroidal anti-inflammatory drugs (NSAIDs): increased risk of hyperkalaemia.
Potassium-sparing diuretics: increased risk of hyperkalaemia.
Thiazide diuretics: increased risk of hypokalaemia (but potassium supplements seldom necessary with small dose of diuretic).

Dose

Mild deficiency, oral, 1500–4000 mg daily, with plenty of fluid (liquid preparations should be diluted well).

As a dietary supplement, no dose has been established.

Prebiotics

Description

Prebiotics are oligosaccharides (polymers of various monosaccharides containing less than 20 sugar units) that are not digestible by human digestive enzymes. These include inulin, oligofructose and fructo-oligosaccharides.

Action

Prebiotics stimulate the numbers and activities of healthy gastrointestinal bacteria, particularly bifidobacteria and lactobacilli. Although prebiotics are not digested in the small intestine they are fermented by bacteria in the colon. They are regarded as a part of dietary fibre.

Dietary sources

The first dietary source consumed is human milk. Some infant formulas also contain prebiotics. They are present in plant foods, principally bananas, onions, asparagus and artichokes.

Possible uses[1–5]

Health effect or disease risk	Strength of evidence
Enhance immune system	P
Reduce cancer risk	I
Enhance mineral absorption	P
Increase resistance to pathogenic bacteria	P
Irritable bowel syndrome	I
Improve blood lipid profile	I
Improve bone formation	I

I, insufficient; P, possible.

Precautions/contraindications

None. Caution in people with altered immune function.

Pregnancy/breastfeeding

No problems known.

Adverse effects

Bloating and flatulence may occur.

Interactions

None reported.

Dose

Not established.

References

1. Osborn DA, Sinn JK. Prebiotics in infants for prevention of allergic disease and food hypersensitivity. *Cochrane Database Syst Rev* 2007(4): CD006474
2. Scholz-Ahrens KE, Ade P, Marten B *et al*. Prebiotics, probiotics, and synbiotics affect mineral absorption, bone mineral content, and bone structure. *J Nutr* 2007; 137(3 suppl 2): S838–S846.
3. Geier MS, Butler RN, Howarth GS. Inflammatory bowel disease: current insights into pathogenesis and new therapeutic options; probiotics, prebiotics and synbiotics. *Int J Food Microbiol* 2007; 115: 1–11.
4. Macfarlane S, Macfarlane GT, Cummings JH. Review article: prebiotics in the gastrointestinal tract. *Aliment Pharmacol Ther* 2006; 24: 701–714.
5. Geier MS, Butler RN, Howarth GS. Probiotics, prebiotics and synbiotics: a role in chemoprevention for colorectal cancer? *Cancer Biol Ther* 2006; 5: 1265–1269.

Probiotics

Description

Probiotics are viable microbial food ingredients that have a beneficial effect on the gastrointestinal tract. Most probiotics are lactobacilli (e.g. *Lactobacillus acidophilus, Lactobacillus reuteri, Lactobacillus bifidus*). They are consumed mainly as fermented dairy products such as yogurts or freeze-dried cultures.

Action

They appear to stimulate immune response and defend against intestinal and food borne pathogens.

Possible uses[1–8]

Health effect or disease risk	Strength of evidence
Reduce duration of acute diarrhoea in children	C
Reduce incidence of acute diarrhoea in adults	P
Prevent travellers' diarrhoea	P
Reduce duration of travellers' diarrhoea	P
Prevent antibiotic-associated diarrhoea	I
Reduce duration of antibiotic-associated diarrhoea	P
Alleviate lactose intolerance	I
Prevent vaginal yeast infections	I
Enhance immune system	P
Improve allergic conditions	P
Lower cholesterol	I
Enhance *Helicobacter pylori* eradication	P
Reduce cancer risk	I

continued

(*continued*)

Reduce symptoms of irritable bowel syndrome (IBS)	P
Reduce symptoms of ulcerative colitis	P
Reduce symptoms of Crohn's disease	I
Food allergy	I
Reduce risk of respiratory infections	I

C, convincing; I, insufficient; P, possible.

Bioavailability

Commercial products do not always contain sufficient viable bacteria.

Precautions/contraindications

None, but caution in immunocompromised patients.

Pregnancy/breastfeeding

No problems reported.

Adverse effects

None.

Interactions

None reported.

Dose

Not established.

References

1. Gill H, Prasad J. Probiotics, immunomodulation, and health benefits. *Adv Exp Med Biol* 2008; 606: 423–454.
2. Zigra PI, Maipa VE, Alamanos YP. Probiotics and remission of ulcerative colitis: a systematic review. *Neth J Med* 2007; 65: 411–418.
3. Franceschi F, Cazzato A, Nista EC *et al*. Role of probiotics in patients with *Helicobacter pylori* infection. *Helicobacter* 2007; 12(suppl 2): 59–63.
4. Borowiec AM, Fedorak RN. The role of probiotics in management of irritable bowel syndrome. *Curr Gastroenterol Rep* 2007; 9: 393–400.

5. Falagas ME, Betsi GI, Athanasiou S. Probiotics for the treatment of women with bacterial vaginosis. *Clin Microbiol Infect* 2007; 13: 657–664.
6. Johnston BC, Supina AL, Ospina M, Vohra S. Probiotics for the prevention of pediatric antibiotic-associated diarrhea. *Cochrane Database Syst Rev* 2007 (2): CD004827
7. Osborn DA, Sinn JK. Probiotics in infants for prevention of allergic disease and food hypersensitivity. *Cochrane Database Syst Rev* 2007(4): CD006474
8. Sazawal S, Hiremath G, Dhingra U, Malik P, Deb S, Black RE. Efficacy of probiotics in prevention of acute diarrhoea: a meta-analysis of masked, randomised, placebo-controlled trials. *Lancet Infect Dis* 2006; 6: 374–382.

Psyllium

Description

Psyllium (ispaghula) is the mucilage obtained from the seed coat (husk or hull) of *Plantago ovata*. It contains a water-soluble, gel-forming polysaccharide and is a rich source of dietary fibre

Action

Stimulates peristalsis, increases stool weight, delays gastric emptying, improves water-absorbing capacity of the faeces, reduces gastric acid production, lowers cholesterol and delays absorption of carbohydrate. It is fermented in the large intestine to form short-chain fatty acids.

Possible uses[1,2]

Health effect or disease risk	Strength of evidence
Improves constipation	C
Improves diarrhoea	C
Lowers cholesterol	C
Improves insulin and glucose control in diabetes	P
Improves symptoms of irritable bowel syndrome (IBS)	I
Improves symptoms of ulcerative colitis	I

C, convincing; I, insufficient; P, possible.

Precautions/contraindications

Gastrointestinal obstruction, swallowing disorders and allergy to psyllium.

Pregnancy/breastfeeding

No problems reported.

Adverse effects

Flatulence, abdominal pain, diarrhoea and nausea. Possibly gastrointestinal obstruction, unless consumed with plenty of water.

Interactions

Drugs

Anti-diabetic drugs: psyllium may lower blood glucose and have an additive effect with anti-diabetic drugs.
Aspirin: absorption may be reduced.
Carbamazepine: absorption may be reduced.
Digoxin: absorption may be reduced.
Lithium: absorption may be reduced.
Statins: psyllium may have an additive effect in reducing blood cholesterol.
Warfarin: theoretical risk of reduced absorption, but clinical studies have not demonstrated an effect.

Nutrients

Minerals and vitamins: psyllium may reduce the absorption of all nutrients (in particular minerals such as calcium, iron, zinc and magnesium).

Dose

Wide ranges of doses have been used in studies, but are not clearly established.

- In constipation, 7–40 g daily in two to three divided doses has been used.
- In cholesterol lowering, the most commonly used doses in adults have ranged from 10 g to 20 g psyllium daily and in children from 5 g to 10 g daily, in two or three divided doses.
- In type 2 diabetes, up to 45 g daily has been given to lower blood glucose.
- For IBS, 6–30 g daily has been used.

For commercial licensed and prescribable preparations of ispaghula, doses can be found in the *British National Formulary*.

Psyllium should always be taken with plenty of fluid and doses avoided just before bedtime (to prevent gastrointestinal obstruction).

References

1. Petchetti L, Frishman WH, Petrillo R, Raju K. Nutriceuticals in cardiovascular disease: psyllium. *Cardiol Rev* 2007; 15: 116–122
2. Singh B. Psyllium as therapeutic and drug delivery agent. *Int J Pharm* 2007; 334: 1–14.

Pumpkin seeds

Description

Pumpkin seeds are the seeds of *Curcubita pepo.*

Constituents

Pumpkin seeds contain 30–50% oil. The main fatty acids are linoleic (*n*-6 polyunsaturated fatty acid), oleic (*n*-9 monounsaturated fatty acid), and the saturated fatty acids palmitic and stearic acids. Pumpkin seeds also contain a small amount of linolenic acid (*n*-3 polyunsaturated fatty acid) and phytosterols. The oil is rich in vitamin E and contains a range of other vitamins and minerals (e.g. vitamin A, B vitamins, magnesium, iron, zinc and copper).

Action

Associated with diuretic, anthelmintic, antihypertensive, anti-diabetic, anti-inflammatory, antioxidant, anti-tumour, hypocholesterolaemic and immunomodulatory activity, ACE inhibitory and α-glucosidase activity, suggesting that pumpkin seeds could reduce the risk of complications linked to hypertension and hyperglycaemia.

Possible uses[1]

Health effect or disease risk	Strength of evidence
Improve symptoms of benign prostatic hyperplasia (BPH)	I
Reduce risk of kidney stones	I
Lower cholesterol	C
Improve insulin and glucose control in diabetes	P
Improve symptoms of irritable bowel syndrome (IBS)	I

C, convincing; I, insufficient; P, possible.

Precautions/contraindications

None known.

Pregnancy/breastfeeding

No harmful effects reported. No long-term data exist on pumpkin seed supplements.

Adverse effects

Allergic reactions.

Interactions

None reported.

Dose

Not established. Supplements generally contain 300–600 mg of pumpkin seed oil. For BPH, pumpkin seed oil, 480 mg in three divided doses has been used.

Reference

1. Caili F, Huan S, Quanhong L. A review on pharmacological activities and utilization technologies of pumpkin. *Plant Foods Hum Nutr* 2006; 61: 73–80.

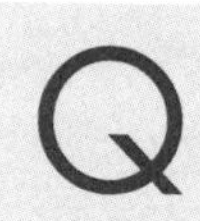

Quercetin

Description

Quercetin (3,3′,4′,5,7-pentahydroxyflavone) is one of the most abundant bioflavonoids in edible fruits and vegetables.

Dietary intake

Estimated intake is 25–50 mg daily.

Action

Quercetin has been shown *in vitro* to:

- Act as an antioxidant.
- Inhibit LDL oxidation.
- Inhibit the nitric oxide pathway.
- Have anti-inflammatory activity, possibly as a result of an influence on the production of eicosanoids, including leukotrienes and prostaglandins, and also cytokines.
- Have potential as an anti-cancer agent through interaction with type II oestrogen-binding sites, inhibition of tyrosine kinase, upregulation of tumour suppressor genes, induction of apoptosis and inhibition of tumour necrosis factor-α.
- Have antihistamine activity.

Dietary sources

Apples; black, green and buckwheat tea; onions (particularly the outer rings); raspberries; red wine; red grapes; cherries; citrus fruits; and broccoli and other green leafy vegetables.

Possible uses[1,2]

Health effect or disease risk	Strength of evidence
Reduces risk of cardiovascular disease	I
Reduces risk of cancer	I
Reduces risk of cataract	I
Management of autoimmune disease	I
Improves symptoms of schizophrenia	I

I, insufficient.

Precautions/contraindications

None reported.

Pregnancy/breastfeeding

No problems have been reported, but there have not been sufficient studies to guarantee the safety of quercetin in pregnancy and breastfeeding.

Adverse effects

Orally, quercetin may cause headache and tingling of the extremities. Mutagenicity has been observed *in vitro* but not *in vivo*.[3]

Interactions

None reported.

Dose

The dose is not established. Typical oral doses range from 400 mg to 500 mg three times daily.

References

1. Perez-Vizcaino F, Duarte J, Andriantsitohaina R. Endothelial function and cardiovascular disease: effects of quercetin and wine polyphenols. *Free Radic Res* 2006; 40: 1054–1065.
2. Lamson DW, Brignall MS. Antioxidants and cancer, part 3: quercetin. *Altern Med Rev* 2000; 5: 196–208.

3. Harwood M, Danielewska-Nikiel B, Borzelleca JF, Flamm GW, Williams GM, Lines TC. A critical review of the data related to the safety of quercetin and lack of evidence of in vivo toxicity, including lack of genotoxic/carcinogenic properties. *Food Chem Toxicol* 2007; 45: 2179–2205.

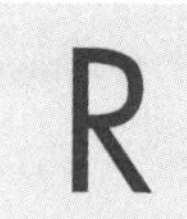

Resveratrol

Description

Resveratrol is a polyphenol, (3,5,4′-trihydroxy-*trans*-stilbene).

Action

Resveratrol has been shown *in vitro* to:

- Have antioxidant activity.
- Inhibit cholesterol synthesis.
- Inhibit atherosclerosis.
- Inhibit LDL oxidation.
- Protect and maintain endothelial tissue.
- Suppress platelet aggregation.
- Promote vasodilatation.
- Defend against ischaemic reperfusion injury.
- Have oestrogenic activity.
- Have anti-cancer activity.

Dietary sources

Skin of grapes and in wine. Red wine has a higher concentration than white wine.

Possible uses[1]

Health effect or disease risk	Strength of evidence
Protect against cardiovascular disease	I

I, insufficient.

Precautions/contraindications

None.

Pregnancy/breastfeeding

No problems reported, but resveratrol may be oestrogenic. Alcohol should not be consumed during pregnancy.

Adverse effects

Resveratrol is similar in structure to diethylstilbestrol (a synthetic oestrogen) and it could have the potential to stimulate breast cancer. More studies are needed.

Interactions

None reported.

Dose

The dose is not established.

Reference

1. Das S, Das DK. Resveratrol: a therapeutic promise for cardiovascular diseases. *Recent Patents Cardiovasc Drug Discov* 2007; 2: 133–138.

Riboflavin

Description

Riboflavin (vitamin B_2) is a water-soluble vitamin of the vitamin B complex.

Human requirements

DRVs for riboflavin							
Age	UK				USA		FAO/ WHO
	LNRI (mg/ day)	EAR (mg/ day)	RNI (mg/ day)	EVM (mg/ day)	RDA (mg/ day)	TUL (mg/ day)	RNI (mg/ day)
0–6 months	0.2	0.3	0.4		0.3	–	0.3
7–12 months	0.2	0.3	0.4		0.4	–	0.4
1–3 years	0.3	0.5	0.6		0.5	–	0.5
4–6 years	0.4	0.6	0.8		–	–	0.6
4–8 years	–	–	–		0.6	–	–
7–10 years	0.5	0.8	1.0		1.2	–	0.9[b]
9–13 years	–	–	–		0.9	–	–
Males							
11–14 years	0.8	1.0	1.2		–	–	1.2[c]
15–18 years	0.8	1.0	1.3		–	–	1.2
19–50+ years	0.8	1.0	1.3		–	–	1.3
14–70+ years				100	1.3	–	–
Females							
11–14 years	0.8	0.9	1.1		–	–	1.0[c]

continued

(continued)

14–18 years 15–50+ years 19–70+ years	 0.8 –	 0.9 –	 1.1 –	 100	1.0 – 1.1	– – –	1.0 1.1 –
Pregnancy	[a]	[a]	+0.3		1.4		1.4
Lactation	–	–	+0.5		1.6	–	1.6

EU RDA = 1.6 mg.
EAR, estimated average requirement; EU RDA, European Union recommended daily allowance; EVM, likely safe daily intake from supplements alone; LNRI, lower reference nutrient intake; RDA, recommended daily allowance; RNI, reference nutrient intake; TUL, tolerable upper intake level.
[a]No increment.
[b]7–9 years.
[c]10–14 years.

Dietary intake

In the UK, the average adult diet provides: for men, 2.11 mg daily; for women, 1.60 mg.

Action

- Functions as a coenzyme in numerous oxidation–reduction reactions.
- An essential component of two flavoprotein coenzymes: flavin mononucleotide (FMN) and flavin adenine dinucleotide (FAD).
- Involved in the activation of vitamin B_6 and conversion of folic acid to its coenzymes.

Dietary sources

Widely distributed in foods but in small amounts. Richest food sources are milk, eggs, meat, poultry, fish, green vegetables (broccoli, spinach and turnip greens) and enriched breakfast cereals.

Possible uses[1,2]

Health effect or disease risk	Strength of evidence
Migraine	P
Lactic acidosis induced by antiretroviral therapy	P

P, possible.

Precautions/contraindications

None reported.

Pregnancy/breastfeeding

No problems reported.

Adverse effects

Riboflavin toxicity is unknown in humans. Large doses may cause yellow discoloration of the urine.

Interactions

Drugs

Alcohol: excessive alcohol intake induces riboflavin deficiency.
Barbiturates: prolonged use may induce riboflavin deficiency.
Oral contraceptives: prolonged use may induce riboflavin deficiency.
Phenothiazines: may increase the requirement for riboflavin.
Probenecid: reduces gastrointestinal absorption and urinary excretion of riboflavin.
Tricyclic antidepressants: may increase the requirement for riboflavin.

Nutrients

Adequate amounts of all B vitamins are required for optimal functioning; deficiency or excess of one B vitamin may lead to abnormalities in the metabolism of another.
Iron: deficiency of riboflavin may impair iron metabolism and produce anaemia.

Dose

Riboflavin is available in the form of tablets and capsules, but is mainly found as a constituent of multivitamin and mineral preparations.

Dietary supplements provide 1–3 mg daily.

References

1. Powers HJ. Riboflavin (vitamin B-2) and health. *Am J Clin Nutr* 2003; 77: 1352–1360.
2. Bianchi A, Salomone S, Caraci F, Pizza V, Bernardini R, D'Amato CC. Role of magnesium, coenzyme Q10, riboflavin, and vitamin B12 in migraine prophylaxis. *Vitam Horm* 2004; 69: 297–312.

Royal jelly

Description

Royal jelly is a yellow–white liquid secreted by the hypopharyngeal glands of 'nurse' worker bees from days 6 to 12 of their adult lives. It is an essential food for the queen bee.

Constituents

Royal jelly contains a mixture of vitamins and minerals. However, a single 500 mg royal jelly capsule contains only 0.2–0.5% of the RNI for each vitamin or mineral.

Action

Royal jelly may have some pharmacological effects, but the only available evidence comes from *in vitro* studies and animal studies. It appears to have anti-tumour effects, improve the efficiency of insulin, have vasodilator activity and exhibit antimicrobial activity.

Possible uses

Many unsubstantiated claims have been made for royal jelly, mainly in the area of rejuvenation and anti-ageing. Recent, preliminary research suggests that royal jelly may have beneficial effects on lipoprotein metabolism[1] and act as an antioxidant.

Precautions/contraindications

Avoid in asthma (adverse effects reported).

Pregnancy/breastfeeding

No problems reported, but there have not been sufficient studies to guarantee the safety of royal jelly in pregnancy and breastfeeding. Royal jelly is probably best avoided.

Adverse effects

Allergic reactions, which can be severe. Life-threatening bronchospasm has occurred in patients with asthma after ingestion of royal jelly. Royal jelly has been responsible for immunoglobulin IgE-mediated anaphylaxis, leading to death in at least one individual. One report of haemorrhagic colitis occurred in a 53-year-old woman after taking royal jelly for 25 days.

Interactions

None reported.

Dose

- Royal jelly is available in the form of tablets and capsules.
- The dose is not established. Dietary supplements provide 250–500 mg daily.

References

1. Guo H, Saiga A, Sato M *et al.* Royal jelly supplementation improves lipoprotein metabolism in humans. *J Nutr Sci Vitaminol (Tokyo)* 2007; 53: 345–348.
2. Nagai T, Inoue R, Suzuki N, Nagashima T. Antioxidant properties of enzymatic hydrolysates from royal jelly. *J Med Food* 2006; 9: 363–367.

S

S-Adenosyl methionine

Description

This is a sulphur-containing amino acid synthesised in the body from the essential amino acid methionine.

Action

S-Adenosyl methionine (SAM) functions mainly as a methyl donor in pathways that lead to the production of DNA and RNA, neurotransmitters and phospholipids. Its involvement in phospholipid synthesis may mean that it has a role in membrane fluidity. SAM is also involved in transulphuration reactions, regulating the formation of the sulphur-containing amino acids, cysteine, glutathione (GSH) and taurine. GSH is an antioxidant, so SAM is proposed to have antioxidant activity

Possible uses[1–3]

Health effect or disease risk	Strength of evidence
Depression	PR
Alcoholic liver disease	I
Osteoarthritis	P
Fibromyalgia	P
Reduces homocysteine	I

I, insufficient; P, possible; PR, probable.

Bioavailability

SAM (1600 mg daily) appears to be significantly bioavailable after an oral dose.[4]

Precautions/contraindications

Avoid in bleeding or haemostatic disorders.

Pregnancy/breastfeeding

No problems reported, but there have been insufficient studies to guarantee the safety of SAM in pregnancy and breastfeeding. SAM is best avoided.

Adverse effects

Minor side effects, including nausea, dry mouth and restlessness, have been occasionally reported.

Interactions

None reported, but in theory SAM could potentiate the activity of antidepressants, anticoagulants and anti-platelet drugs.

Dose

The dose is not established. Studies have used doses of 400–1600 mg daily.

References

1. Papakostas GI, Alpert JE, Fava M. *S*-Adenosyl-methionine in depression: a comprehensive review of the literature. *Curr Psychiatry Rep* 2003; 5: 460–466.
2. Rambaldi A, Gluud C. *S*-Adenosyl-L-methionine for alcoholic liver diseases. *Cochrane Database Syst Rev* 2006(2): CD002235.
3. Hardy ML, Coulter I, Morton SC *et al*. *S*-Adenosyl-L-methionine for treatment of depression, osteoarthritis, and liver disease. *Evid Rep Technol Assess (Summ)* 2003(64): 1–3.
4. Goren JL, Stoll AL, Damico KE, Sarmiento IA, Cohen BM. Bioavailability and lack of toxicity of S-adenosyl-L-methionine (SAMe) in humans. *Pharmacotherapy* 2004; 24: 1501–1507.

Selenium

Description

Selenium is an essential trace element.

Human requirements

DRVs for selenium							
Age	UK			USA			FAO/ WHO
	LRNI (mcg/ day)	RNI (mcg/ day)	EVM (mcg/ day)	RDA (mcg/ day)	AI (mcg/ day)	TUL (mcg/ day)	RNI (mcg/ day)
0–3 months	4	10		–	15	45	6
4–6 months	5	13		–	15	45	6
7–9 months	5	10		–	20	45	10
10–12 months	6	10		–	20	45	10
1–3 years	7	15		20		90	17
4–6 years	10	20			–	–	22
4–8 years	–	–	–	30		150	–
7–10 years	16	30		–		–	21[b]
Males							
11–14 years	25	45		40		400	32[c]
15–18 years	40	70		50		400	32
19–50+ years	40	75	200	70		400	34[d]
Females							
11–14 years	25	45		45		400	26[c]

continued

(continued)

15–18 years	40	60		50		400	26
19–50+ years	40	60	200	55		400	26[e]
Pregnancy	[a]	[a]		65		400	28–30
Lactation	+15	+15		75		400	35–42

EU RDA = none.

AI, adequate intake; EU RDA, European Union recommended daily allowance; EVM, likely safe daily intake from supplements alone; LNRI, lower reference nutrient intake; RDA, recommended daily allowance; RNI, reference nutrient intake; TUL, tolerable upper intake level.

[a]No increment.

[b]7–9 years.

[c]10–14 years.

[d]>65 years, 33 mcg/day.

[e]51–65 years, 26 mcg/day; >65 years, 25 mcg/day.

Dietary intake

In the UK, the average adult diet provides 39 mcg daily.

Action

A major antioxidant nutrient, selenium protects cell membranes, preserves tissue elasticity, and slows down the hardening of tissues by preventing free radical generation from oxidant damage. It functions as a component of enzymes involved in thyroid hormone metabolism and immune system function. Interacts with vitamin E; a deficiency in vitamin E can be partially corrected by selenium and vice versa.

Dietary sources

Seafood, meat, liver and whole grains are good sources. Fruit and vegetables are relatively poor sources.

Possible uses[1-6]

Health effect or disease risk	Strength of evidence
Protects against cancer overall	I
Protects against prostate cancer	P
Reduces risk of CVD	I

Enhances immunity	I
Improves mood	I
Improves rheumatoid arthritis	I
Adjunct in asthma	I

I, insufficient; P, possible.

Bioavailability

Organic selenomethionine and organic selenium yeast have a higher bioavailability than inorganic preparations (e.g. sodium selenite).

Precautions/contraindications

Yeast-containing selenium products should be avoided by patients taking monoamine oxidase inhibitors (MAOIs).

Pregnancy/breastfeeding

No problems with normal intakes.

Adverse effects

There is a narrow margin of safety for selenium. Adverse effects include hair loss, nail changes, skin lesions, nausea, diarrhoea, irritability, metallic taste, garlic-smelling breath, fatigue and peripheral neuropathy.

Interactions

There is some evidence that clozapine may reduce selenium levels and this could be important in the pathogenesis of cardiac side effects with clozapine.

Dose

Selenium is available mainly in 'antioxidant' supplements with vitamins E and A, and is also an ingredient in multivitamin supplements.

The dose is not established; 50–100 mcg daily is considered to be safe.

References

1. Rayman MP. Selenium in cancer prevention: a review of the evidence and mechanism of action. *Proc Nutr Soc* 2005; 64: 527–542.

2. Rayman M, Thompson A, Warren-Perry M *et al.* Impact of selenium on mood and quality of life. *Biol Psychiatry* 2006; 59: 147–154.
3. Dodig S, Cepelak I. The facts and controversies about selenium. *Acta Pharm* 2004; 54: 261–276.
4. Combs GF, Jr. Status of selenium in prostate cancer prevention. *Br J Cancer* 2004; 91: 195–199.
5. Allam MF, Lucane RA. Selenium supplementation for asthma. *Cochrane Database Syst Rev* 2004(2): CD003538.
6. Alissa EM, Bahijri SM, Ferns GA. The controversy surrounding selenium and cardiovascular disease: a review of the evidence. *Med Sci Monit* 2003; 9: RA9–RA18.

Shark cartilage

Description

This is cartilage obtained from various types of shark. It contains a mixture of glycosaminoglycans (including chondroitin sulphate). Also thought to contain anti-angiogenesis factors, which inhibit the growth of new blood vessels, typically seen in malignant tumours; this mechanism could, in theory, be helpful in human cancer.

Action

Thought to have an anti-tumour effect due to anti-angiogenesis factors.

Possible uses[1]

Health effect or disease risk	Strength of evidence
Reduces risk of cancer	I

I, insufficient.

Precautions/contraindications

Avoid in patients with hepatic disease. There has been a single case report of hepatitis attributed to shark cartilage.

Pregnancy/breastfeeding

There are no available data. Shark cartilage should be avoided.

Adverse effects

Hepatitis and various gastrointestinal effects (e.g. nausea, vomiting, constipation) have been reported. A case study has found that shark cartilage dust can be a cause of asthma. A 38-year-old man reported chest symptoms at work in association with exposure to shark cartilage dust and was diagnosed with asthma. Six months later he complained of shortness of breath and died from asthma confirmed *post mortem*.

Interactions

None reported.

Dose

- Shark cartilage is available in the form of tablets, capsules and powder.
- The dose is not established.
- There is no proven value of shark cartilage supplements.

Reference

1. Gonzalez RP, Leyva A, Moraes MO. Shark cartilage as source of antiangiogenic compounds: from basic to clinical research. *Biol Pharm Bull* 2001; 241: 1097–1101.

Silicon

Description

An essential trace element in animals; possibly essential in humans but not proven.

Human requirements

Not established. The Food Standards Agency's (FSA's) Expert Vitamins and Minerals (EVM) group set a safe upper level for adults for total silicon intake (from foods and supplements) of 760 mg daily.

Dietary intake

Intake in the UK is unknown. Intakes in the USA range from 20 mg to 50 mg daily.

Action

It is believed to function in the metabolism of connective tissue, formation of collagen, calcification of bones and maintenance of elastic tissue integrity.

Dietary sources

Found in many foods especially unrefined grains, cereal products and root vegetables. Animal foods are low in silicon.

Possible uses[1]

Health effect or disease risk	Strength of evidence
Reduces risk of CVD	I
Reduces risk of osteoporosis	I

continued

(*continued*)

Reduces risk of osteoarthritis	I
Reduces risk of hypertension	I
Reduces risk of Alzheimer's disease	I

I, insufficient.

Precautions/contraindications

No at-risk groups or situations have been documented.

Pregnancy/breastfeeding

No problems have been reported, but there have been insufficient studies to guarantee the safety of silicon in pregnancy and breastfeeding.

Adverse effects

There are few data on the oral toxicity of silicon in humans. In humans, adverse effects are primarily limited to silicosis, a lung disease resulting from the inhalation of silica particles.

Interactions

Drugs

None reported.

Nutrients

Silicon has been reported to interact with a number of minerals, including aluminium, copper and zinc.

Dose

The dose is not established. Dietary supplements in the UK provide doses of up to 500 mg daily.

Reference

1. Jugdaohsingh R. Silicon and bone health. *J Nutr Health Aging* 2007; 11: 99–110.

Spirulina

Description

Spirulina is a blue–green microscopic alga.

Action

Spirulina consists of approximately 65–70% crude protein, high concentration of B vitamins, phenylalanine, iron and other minerals. However, all the B vitamins (including B_{12}) are thought to be in the form of analogues and nutritionally insignificant. The iron is believed to be highly bioavailable with 1.5–2 mg being absorbed from a 10 g dose of spirulina.

Possible uses[1]

Health effect or disease risk	Strength of evidence
Lipid lowering	I
Reduces blood glucose	I
Protects against allergic rhinitis	I
Protects against Alzheimer's disease	I
Protects against peptic ulcer	I
Anti-ageing	I

I, insufficient.

Precautions/contraindications

Spirulina may be contaminated with mercury.

Pregnancy/breastfeeding

Avoid (contaminants – see Precautions/contraindications).

Adverse effects

Effects not known (contaminants – see Precautions/contraindications).

Interactions

None known.

Dose

- Spirulina is available in the form of tablets, capsules and powders.
- The dose is not established. There is no proven benefit of spirulina. Dietary supplements provide 6–10 g per daily dose.

Reference

1. Khan Z, Bhadouria P, Bisen PS. Nutritional and therapeutic potential of Spirulina. *Curr Pharm Biotechnol* 2005; 6: 373–379.

Superoxide dismutase

Description

This is a group of enzymes that is widely distributed in the body; several different forms exist with varying metal content (e.g. copper and zinc). Copper-containing superoxide dismutase (SOD) is extracellular and present in high concentrations in the lungs, thyroid and uterus, and in small amounts in plasma. SOD containing copper and zinc is present within the cells and found in high concentrations in the brain, erythrocytes, kidney, liver, pituitary and thyroid.

Action

SOD enzymes act as scavengers of superoxide radicals and protect against oxidative damage (by catalysing conversion of superoxide radicals to peroxide).

Possible uses[1]

Health effect or disease risk	Strength of evidence
Prevents CVD	I
Prevents cancer	I
Retards ageing	I

I, insufficient.

Precautions/contraindications

None reported.

Pregnancy/breastfeeding

No problems reported, but there have been insufficient studies to guarantee the safety of SOD in pregnancy and breastfeeding.

Adverse effects

None reported from oral doses.

Interactions

None reported.

Dose

SOD is available in the form of tablets and capsules. However, products may not have any of the stated activity because they are acid labile and break down before absorption.

The dose is not established. Not recommended as a dietary supplement (probably ineffective).

Reference

1. Noor R, Mittal S, Iqbal J. Superoxide dismutase – applications and relevance to human diseases. *Med Sci Monit* 2002; 8: RA210–RA215.

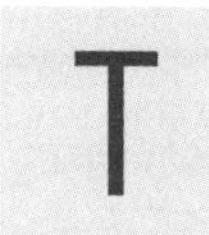

Thiamine

Description

Thiamine (vitamin B_1) is a water-soluble vitamin of the vitamin B complex.

Human requirements

DRVs for thiamine								
Age	UK					USA		FAO/ WHO
	LNRI (mg/ 1000 kcal)	EAR (mg/ 1000 kcal)	RNI (mg/ 1000 kcal)	RNI (mg/ day)	EVM	RDA (mg/ day)	TUL (mg/ day)	RNI (mg/ day)
0–6 months	0.2	0.23	0.3	0.2		0.2	–	0.2
7–12 months	0.2	0.23	0.3	0.3		0.3	–	0.3
1–3 years	0.23	0.3	0.4	0.5		0.5	–	0.5
4–6 years	0.23	0.3	0.4	0.7		0.7	–	0.6
4–8 years						0.6		
7–10 years	0.23	0.3	0.4	0.7		–	0.9[a]	
9–13 years				0.9	–	–		

continued

(continued)

Males								
11–14 years	0.23	0.3	0.4	0.9			–	1.2[b]
15–50 years	0.23	0.3	0.4	0.9	100 (mg/day)		–	1.2
14–70+ years					1.2			
Females								
11–14 years	0.23	0.3	0.4	0.7			–	1.1[b]
14–18 years						1.0	–	–
15–50+ years	0.23	0.3	0.4	0.8	100 (mg/day)		–	1.1
19–70+ years						1.1	–	–
Pregnancy	0.23	0.3	0.4	+0.1[c]		1.4	–	+0.1
Lactation	0.23	0.3	0.4	+0.2		1.5	–	+0.2

EU RDA = 1.6 mg.

EAR, estimated average requirement; EU RDA, European Union recommended daily allowance; EVM, likely safe daily intake from supplements alone; LNRI, lower reference nutrient intake; RDA, recommended daily allowance; RNI, reference nutrient intake; TUL, tolerable upper intake level.

[a] 7–9 years.

[b] 10–14 years.

[c] Last trimester only.

Dietary intake

In the UK, the average adult diet provides: for men, 2.0 mg daily; for women, 1.54 mg.

Action

Thiamine functions as a coenzyme in the metabolism of carbohydrates and branched-chain amino acids. It helps normal nervous system activity and gastrointestinal tract muscle tone.

Dietary sources

Brewers' yeast, unrefined or enriched cereals, bran cereals, liver and kidney, lean pork, legumes and nuts. Cooking losses are high if cooking water is discarded or during prolonged heating at high temperatures.

Possible uses[1]

Health effect or disease risk	Strength of evidence
Alzheimer's disease	I
Mouth ulcers	I
Insect repellent	P
Alcoholism	C

C, convincing; I, insufficient; P, possible.

Bioavailability

Thiamine is generally bioavailable. No robust data on supplements.

Precautions/contraindications

Known hypersensitivity to thiamine.

Pregnancy/breastfeeding

No problems reported.

Adverse effects

No toxic effects (except possibly gastric upset) with high oral doses. Large parenteral doses are generally well tolerated, but there have been rare reports of anaphylactic reactions (coughing, difficulty in breathing and swallowing, flushing, skin rash, swelling of face, lips and eyelids).

Interactions

Drugs

Alcohol: excessive alcohol intake induces thiamine deficiency.
Furosemide: may increase urinary loss of thiamine;[2] prolonged furosemide therapy may induce thiamine deficiency; thiamine supplementation (200 mg daily) has been shown to improve left ventricular function in patients with congestive heart failure receiving furosemide therapy.

Nutrients

Adequate amounts of all B vitamins are required for optimal functioning; deficiency or excess of one B vitamin may lead to abnormalities in the metabolism of another.

Dose

Thiamine is available in the form of tablets and capsules. It is also found in multivitamins and in brewers' yeast supplements.

No benefit of a dose beyond the RDA (as a food supplement) has been established.

Doses for mild and severe deficiency can be found in the *British National Formulary*. The dose for prophylaxis or treatment of Wernicke–Korsakoff syndrome caused by alcohol abuse, and the length of time that thiamine should be given after drinking has ceased, have not been clarified.

References

1. Monograph Thiamine. *Altern Med Rev* 2003; 8: 59–62.
2. Sica DS. Loop diuretic therapy, thiamine balance, and heart failure. *Congest Heart Fail* 2007;13: 244–247.

Tin

Description

Tin is a metallic element usually found in the form of the dioxide (SnO_2).

Human requirements

Tin has not been shown to be essential in humans. No British DRVs. The FSA's EVM group stated that intake of tin of up to 0.22 mg/kg body weight per day (equivalent to 13 mg tin daily in a 60 kg adult) would not be expected to have any harmful effects but did not set a safe upper level or guidance level for adults for supplemental tin intake.

Intake

Mean intake of dietary tin in the UK is 1.8 mg daily, with an estimated maximum intake of 6.3 mg daily.

Action

The actions of dietary tin are not known. However, it is thought that it may function as part of metalloenzymes.

Dietary sources

Tin intake is essentially dependent on food stored in tin cans. The main dietary sources of tin are tinned vegetables and fruit products. The presence of tin in fresh food is highly dependent on the soil concentration of tin. Stannous chloride is a permitted food additive (E512).

Bioavailability

Bioavailability varies and depends on the oxidation state of the tin salt.

Possible uses

No beneficial human health effects from consuming dietary tin are known. Tin has been claimed to have immune-enhancing properties in animals, but there is no evidence that tin has these effects in humans.

Precautions/contraindications

None reported.

Pregnancy/breastfeeding

No problems have been reported, but there have not been sufficient studies to guarantee the safety of tin in pregnancy and breastfeeding.

Adverse effects

Acute tin poisoning (from food or drinks) is associated with gastrointestinal effects (cramps, vomiting, nausea and diarrhoea), headaches and chills.

Interactions

None reported.

Dose

The dose is not established. Supplements in the UK contain up to 10 mcg in a daily dose.

Reference

1. Food Standards Agency. *Risk Assessment. Tin.* Available at www.eatwell.gov.uk/healthydiet/nutritionessentials/vitaminsandminerals/tin (accessed 8 July 2006).

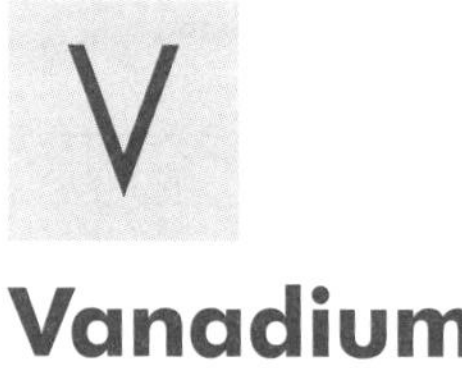

Vanadium

Description

Vanadium is a trace element.

Human requirements

Not established. Vanadium has not been shown to be essential in human beings. There are no DRVs. It is thought that 10 mcg daily is adequate. The US Food and Nutrition Board set a TUL of 1.8 mg daily in adult men and women from the age of 19 years.

Dietary intake

The intake of dietary vanadium in the UK averages 13 mcg daily.[1] Intakes in the USA range from 10 mcg to 60 mcg daily.

Action

Vanadium has no defined function in human beings. It stimulates proliferation of cells and inhibits ATPases and phosphatases. It may have a role in the regulation of the Na^+ pump and the metabolism of bones, glucose and lipids.

Dietary sources

Present in small amounts in most foods, especially mushrooms, shellfish, parsley and dill seed.

Possible uses (pharmacological doses)[1,2]

Health effect or disease risk	Strength of evidence
Lowers cholesterol	P
Lowers triglycerides	P
Improves insulin sensitivity	P
Reduces plasma glucose	P
Ergogenic acid	I

I, insufficient; P, possible.

Bioavailability

Only about 5% of ingested vanadium is absorbed.

Precautions/contraindications

See Adverse effects.

Pregnancy/breastfeeding

No problems reported, but safety studies have not been conducted.

Adverse effects

Vanadium causes abdominal cramps, diarrhoea, haemolysis, increased blood pressure and fatigue. The primary toxic effect in humans occurs from inhaling vanadium dust in industrial settings. This is characterised by rhinitis, wheezing, conjunctivitis, cough, sore throat and chest pain.

Interactions

None reported.

Dose

The dose is not established. Food supplements in the UK provide up to 25 mcg in a daily dose

References

1. Coderre L, Srivastava AK. Vanadium and the cardiovascular functions. *Can J Physiol Pharmacol* 2004; 82: 833–839.

2. Thompson KH, Orvig C. Vanadium in diabetes: 100 years from Phase 0 to Phase I. *J Inorg Biochem* 2006; 100: 1925–1935.

Vitamin A

Description

Vitamin A is a fat-soluble vitamin. Vitamin A is a generic term used to describe compounds that exhibit the biological activity of retinol. The two main components in food are retinol and the carotenoids (see Carotenoids).

Human requirements

DRVs for vitamin A							
Age	UK				USA		FAO/ WHO
	LNRI (mcg retinol equivalent/ day)	EAR (mcg retinol equivalent/ day)	RNI (mcg retinol equivalent/ day)	EVM (mcg retinol equivalent/ day)	RDA (mcg retinol equivalent/ day)	TUL (mcg retinol equivalent/ day)	RNI (mcg retinol equivalent/ day)
0–6 months	150	250	350		400[c]	600	375
7–12 months	150	250	350		500[c]	600	400
1–3 years	200	300	400		300	600	400
4–6 years	200	300	400		–	–	450
4–8 years	–	–	–		400	900	–
7–10 years	250	350	500		–	–	500[a]
9–13 years	–	–	–		600	1700	–
Males 11–14 years	250	400	600		–	–	600[b]

14–18 years	–	–	–		900	2800	600
15–50+ years	300	500	700	1500	–	–	600
19–70+ years	–	–	–		900	3000	–
65+years							600
Females							
11–14 years	250	400	600	1500	–	–	600[b]
14–18 years	–	–	–		700	2800	600
15–50+ years	250	400	250		700	3000	500
19–70+ years	–	–	–		700		
65+years							600
Pregnancy			+100		770[d]	3000[e]	800
Lactation			+350		1300[f]	3000[f]	850

EU RDA = 800 mcg.

EAR, estimated average requirement; EU RDA, European Union recommended daily allowance; EVM, likely safe daily intake from supplements alone; LNRI, lower reference nutrient intake; RDA, recommended daily allowance; RNI, reference nutrient intake; TUL, tolerable upper intake level.

[a]7–9 years.

[b]10–14 years.

[c]Adequate intakes (AIs).

[d]Aged <18 years, 750 mcg.

[e]Aged >18 years, 2800 mcg.

[f]Aged <18 years, 1200 mcg.

Dietary intake

In the UK, the average adult diet provides (retinol equivalents): for men, 911 mcg daily; for women, 671 mcg.

Action

It is necessary for normal growth and development, maintenance of normal epithelial tissue structure, integrity of the immune system, gene regulation, vision and reproduction.

Dietary sources

Fish liver oils, liver and kidney, egg yolk and fortified milk.

Possible uses

Health effect or disease risk	Strength of evidence
Prevention and treatment of vitamin A deficiency	C
Reduces risk of cancer	I

C, convincing; I, insufficient.

Precautions/contraindications

Pregnancy.

Pregnancy/breastfeeding

Caution: excessive doses can be teratogenic. The Department of Health advises avoidance of vitamin A supplements in pregnancy.

Adverse effects[1]

Excessive intake causes headache, dry skin, loss of hair, softening of bones and liver damage. A high incidence of spontaneous abortions and birth defects has been observed in women taking high doses of isotretinoin during the first trimester of pregnancy. Vitamin A intakes above the safe upper level may pose risks to bone health (i.e. reduced bone mineral density and increased risk of hip fracture).

Interactions

Drugs

Anticoagulants: large doses of vitamin A (> 750 mcg, 2500 units) may induce a hypoprothrombinaemic response.
Colestyramine and colestipol: may reduce intestinal absorption of vitamin A.
Colchicine: may reduce intestinal absorption of vitamin A.
Liquid paraffin: may reduce intestinal absorption of vitamin A.
Neomycin: may reduce intestinal absorption of vitamin A.
Retinoids (acitrecin, etretinate, isotretinoin, tretinoin): concurrent administration of vitamin A may result in additive toxic effects.
Statins: prolonged therapy with statins may increase serum vitamin A levels.
Sucralfate: may reduce intestinal absorption of vitamin A.

Nutrients

Iron: in vitamin A deficiency, plasma iron levels fall.
Vitamin C: under conditions of hypervitaminosis A, tissue levels of vitamin C may be reduced and urinary excretion of vitamin C increased; vitamin C may ameliorate the toxic effects of vitamin A.
Vitamin E: large doses of vitamin A increase the need for vitamin E; vitamin E protects against the oxidative destruction of vitamin A.
Vitamin K: under conditions of hypervitaminosis A, hypothrombinaemia may occur; it can be corrected by administration of vitamin K.

Dose

Vitamin A supplementation is not normally required in the UK.

Therapeutic doses may be given but only under medical supervision, e.g. in cystic fibrosis, doses of 1200–3300 mcg (4000–10 000 units) daily may be given.

Reference

1. Penniston KL, Tanumihardjo SA. The acute and chronic toxic effects of vitamin A. *Am J Clin Nutr* 2006; 83: 191–201.

Vitamin B_6

Description

Vitamin B_6 is a water-soluble member of the vitamin B complex. Vitamin B_6 describes the compounds that exhibit the biological activity of pyridoxine. It occurs in food as pyridoxine, pyridoxal and pyridoxamine, so the term 'pyridoxine' is not synonymous with the generic term 'vitamin B_6'.

Human requirements

DRVs for vitamin B_6

Age	UK					USA		FAO/ WHO
	LNRI (mcg/g protein)	EAR (mg/ day)	RNI (mcg/g protein)	RNI (mg/ day)	EVM (mg/ day)	RDA (mg/ day)	TUL (mg/ day)	RNI (mg/ day)
0–6 months	3.5	6	8	0.2		0.1[d]	–	0.1
7–9 months	6	8	10	0.3		0.3[d]	–	0.3
10–12 months	8	10	13	0.4		0.3	–	0.3
1–3 years	8	10	13	0.7		0.5	30	0.5
4–6 years	8	10	13	0.9		–	–	0.6
4–8 years	–	–	–	–		0.6	40	–
7–10 years	8	10	13	1.0		–	–	1.0[b]
9–13 years						1.0	60	–
Males 11–14 years	11	13	15	1.2		–	–	1.3[c]

14–18 years						1.3	80	1.3
15–18 years	11	13	15	1.4				–
19–50+ years	11	13	15	1.4	10	1.3	100	1.3
51–70+ years	–	–	–	–	10	1.7	100	1.7
Females								
11–14 years	11	13	15	1.0		–	–	1.2[c]
14–18 years	–	–	–	–		1.2	80	1.2
15–18 years	11	13	15	1.2		–	–	–
19–50+ years	11	13	15	1.2	10	1.3	100	1.3
51–70+ years	–	–	–	–	10	1.5	100	1.5
Pregnancy	[a]	[a]	[a]	[a]		1.9	100[e]	1.9
Lactation	[a]	[a]	[a]	[a]		2.0	100[e]	2.0

EU RDA = 2 mg.

EAR, estimated average requirement; EU RDA, European Union recommended daily allowance; EVM, likely safe daily intake from supplements alone; LNRI, lower reference nutrient intake; RDA, recommended daily allowance; RNI, reference nutrient intake; TUL, tolerable upper intake level.

[a]No increment.

[b]7–9 years.

[c]10–14 years.

[d]Adequate intakes (AIs).

[e]≤18 years = 80 mg.

Dietary intake

In the UK, the average adult daily diet provides: for men, 2.9 mg; for women, 2.0 mg.

Action

It functions as coenzymes in the metabolism of amino acids, and is also involved in the conversion of tryptophan to nicotinic acid, urea production, metabolism of essential fatty acid and steroid hormone activity.

Dietary sources

It is found in all plant and animal foods. Good sources include muscle meats, liver, pork, egg, whole grain cereals and soya beans.

Possible uses[1–6]

Health effect or disease risk	Strength of evidence
Relieves carpal tunnel syndrome	P
Relieves symptoms of PMS	P
Reduces risk of CVD	P
Reduces symptoms of asthma	I
Treats autism	I
Reduces diabetic neuropathy	P
Improves cognitive function	I

I, insufficient; P, possible.

Bioavailability

Vitamin B_6 is significantly bioavailable.

Precautions/contraindications

Hypersensitivity to pyridoxine.

Pregnancy/breastfeeding

No problems reported with normal intakes. Large doses may result in pyridoxine dependency in infants.

Adverse effects

Large doses (usually >500 mg/day): peripheral neuropathy; unsteady gait; numbness and tingling in feet and hands; loss of limb reflexes; impaired or absent tendon reflexes; photosensitivity on exposure to sun; dizziness; nausea; breast tenderness; and exacerbation of acne.

Interactions

Drugs

Alcohol: increases turnover of pyridoxine.
Cycloserine: may cause anaemia or peripheral neuritis by acting as a pyridoxine antagonist.

Hydralazine: may cause anaemia or peripheral neuritis by acting as a pyridoxine antagonist.
Isoniazid: may cause anaemia or peripheral neuritis by acting as a pyridoxine antagonist.
Levodopa: effects of levodopa are reversed by pyridoxine (even doses as low as 5 mg daily); vitamin B_6 supplements should be avoided; interaction does not occur with co-beneldopa or co-careldopa.
Oestrogens: (including oral contraceptives) may increase requirement for vitamin B_6.
Penicillamine: may cause anaemia or peripheral neuritis by acting as a pyridoxine antagonist.
Theophylline: may increase requirement for vitamin B_6.

Nutrients

Adequate amounts of all B vitamins are required for optimal functioning; deficiency or excess of one B vitamin may lead to abnormalities in the metabolism of another.
Vitamin C: deficiency of vitamin B_6 may lead to vitamin C deficiency.

Dose

As a dietary supplement, 2–5 mg daily.

References

1. Ryan-Harshman M, Aldoori W. Carpal tunnel syndrome and vitamin B_6. *Can Fam Physician* 2007; 53: 1161–1162.
2. Spinneker A, Sola R, Lemmen V, Castillo MJ, Pietrzik K, Gonzalez-Gross M. Vitamin B_6 status, deficiency and its consequences–an overview. *Nutr Hosp* 2007; 22: 7–24.
3. Balk EM, Raman G, Tatsioni A, Chung M, Lau J, Rosenberg IH. Vitamin B_6, B_{12}, and folic acid supplementation and cognitive function: a systematic review of randomized trials. *Arch Intern Med* 2007; 167: 21–30.
4. Nye C, Brice A. Combined vitamin B_6-magnesium treatment in autism spectrum disorder. *Cochrane Database Syst Rev* 2005(4): CD003497.
5. Malouf R, Grimley Evans J. The effect of vitamin B_6 on cognition. *Cochrane Database Syst Rev* 2003(4): CD004393.
6. Kashanian M, Mazinani R, Jalalmanesh S. Pyridoxine (vitamin B_6) therapy for premenstrual syndrome. *Int J Gynecol Obstet* 2007; 96: 43–44.

Vitamin B_{12}

Description

Vitamin B_{12} (cobalamin) is a water-soluble member of the vitamin B complex.

Human requirements

DRVs for vitamin B_{12}							
Age	UK				USA		FAO/ WHO
	LNRI (mcg/ day)	EAR (mcg/ day)	RNI (mcg/ day)	EVM (mcg/ day)	RDA (mcg/ day)	TUL (mcg/ day)	RNI (mcg/ day)
0–6 months	0.1	0.25	0.3		0.4	–	0.4
7–12 months	0.25	0.35	0.4		0.5	–	0.5
1–3 years	0.3	0.4	0.5		0.9	–	0.9
4–6 years	0.5	0.7	0.8			–	1.2
4–8 years					1.2	–	–
7–10 years	0.6	0.8	1.0		–	–	1.8[b]
9–13 years					1.8	–	–
Males							
11–14 years	0.8	1.0	1.2		–	–	2.4[c]
15–50+ years	1.0	1.25	1.5	1000	–	–	2.4
14–70+ years					2.4	–	–
Females							
11–14 years	0.8	1.0	1.2		–	–	2.4[c]

15–50+ years	1.0	1.25	1.5	1000	–	–	2.4
14–70+ years					2.4	–	–
Pregnancy		[a]			2.6	–	2.6
Lactation		+0.5			2.8	–	2.8

EU RDA = 1 mcg.

EAR, estimated average requirement; EU RDA, European Union recommended daily allowance; EVM, likely safe daily intake from supplements alone; LNRI, lower reference nutrient intake; RDA, recommended daily allowance; RNI, reference nutrient intake; TUL, tolerable upper intake level.

[a]No increment.

[b]7–9 years.

[c]10–14 years.

Dietary intake

In the UK, the average adult daily diet provides: for men, 6.5 mcg; for women, 4.8 mcg.

Action

It functions: as a coenzyme in the metabolism of fatty acids and in methyl transfer; in the stimulation of red blood cell formation, function of nervous tissue, synthesis of nucleic acids and nucleoproteins; metabolism of folate and sulphur-containing amino acids

Dietary sources

Present only in animal foods; plant foods are practically devoid of the vitamin. Good food sources are liver, eggs, meat, fish and milk.

Possible uses[1–3]

Health effect or disease risk	Strength of evidence
Prevention or treatment in vitamin B_{12} deficiency (e.g. vegans, older people)	C
Reduces risk of CVD	P
Reduces risk of dementia	I
Treats multiple sclerosis	P

continued

(*continued*)

Sleep disorders	I
Improves diabetic neuropathy	I
Mouth ulcers	I

C, convincing; I, insufficient; P, possible.

Precautions/contraindications

Vitamin B_{12} should not be given for treatment of deficiency until the diagnosis has been fully established (administration of > 10 mcg daily may produce a haematological response in patients with folate deficiency).

Pregnancy/breastfeeding

No problems reported with normal intakes.

Adverse effects

Vitamin B_{12} may occasionally cause diarrhoea and itching skin. Signs of polycythaemia vera may be unmasked. Megadoses may exacerbate acne.

Interactions

Drugs

Alcohol: excessive intake may reduce the absorption of vitamin B_{12}.
Aminoglycosides: may reduce the absorption of vitamin B_{12}.
Aminosalicylates: may reduce the absorption of vitamin B_{12}.
Antibiotics: may interfere with microbiological assay for serum and erythrocyte vitamin B_{12} (false low results).
Chloramphenicol: may reduce the absorption of vitamin B_{12}.
Colestyramine: may reduce the absorption of vitamin B_{12}.
Colchicine: may reduce the absorption of vitamin B_{12}.
Histamine H_2-receptor antagonists: may reduce the absorption of vitamin B_{12}.
Metformin: may reduce the absorption of vitamin B_{12}.
Methyldopa: may reduce the absorption of vitamin B_{12}.
Nitrous oxide: prolonged nitrous oxide anaesthesia inactivates vitamin B_{12}.
Oral contraceptives: may reduce blood levels of vitamin B_{12}.
Potassium chloride (modified release): prolonged administration may reduce the absorption of vitamin B_{12}.
Proton-pump inhibitors: long-term therapy may reduce serum vitamin B_{12} levels.

Nutrients

Folic acid: large doses given continuously may reduce vitamin B_{12} in blood.
Vitamin C: may destroy vitamin B_{12} (avoid large doses of vitamin C within 1 h of oral vitamin B_{12}).

Dose

As a supplement, 2–25 mcg daily.

References

1. Reynolds E. Vitamin B_{12}, folic acid, and the nervous system. *Lancet Neurol* 2006; 5: 949–960.
2. Balk EM, Raman G, Tatsioni A, Chung M, Lau J, Rosenberg IH. Vitamin B_6, B_{12}, and folic acid supplementation and cognitive function: a systematic review of randomized trials. *Arch Intern Med* 2007; 167: 21–30.
3. Wedman-St Louis B. Vitamin B_{12}. A review. *Nephrol News Issues* 2004; 18: 49–51.

Vitamin C

Description

Vitamin C (ascorbic acid) is a water-soluble vitamin.

Human requirements

Smokers have increased requirements.

DRVs for vitamin C									
Age	UK				USA				FAO/ WHO
	LNRI (mg/ day)	EAR (mg/ day)	RNI (mg/ day)	EVM (mg/ day)	EAR (mg/ day)	RDA (mg/ day)	AI (mg/ day)	TUL (mg/ day)	RNI (mg/ day)
0–6 months	6	15	25		–	–	40	–	25
7–12 months	6	15	25		–	–	50	–	30
1–3 years	8	20	30		13	–	–	400	30
4–6 years	8	20	30		–	–	–	–	30
4–8 years	–	–	–		22	25	–	–	650
7–10 years	8	20	30		–	–	–	–	35[a]
9–13 years	–	–	–		39	45	–	1200	40
Males									
11–14 years	9	22	35		–	–	–	–	40[b]
14–18 years	–	–	–		63	75	–	1800	40

15–50 +years	10	25	40	1000	–	–	–	–	–
19–70 +years	–	–	–		75	90	–	2000	45
Females									
11–14 years	9	22	35		–	–	–	–	40
14–18 years	–	–	–		56	65	–	1800	40
15–50 +years	10	25	40	1000	–	–	–	–	–
19–70 +years	–	–	–		60	75	–	2000	45
Preg-nancy	–	–	+10		66[c]/ 70[d]	80[c]/ 85[d]		1800[c]/ 2000[d]	55
Lacta-tion	–	–	+30		96[c]/ 100[d]	115[c]/ 120[d]	1800[c]/ 2000[d]	70	

EU RDA (for labelling purposes) = 60 mg.
EAR, estimated average requirement; EU RDA, European Union recommended daily allowance; EVM, likely safe daily intake from supplements alone; LNRI, lower reference nutrient intake; RDA, recommended daily allowance; RNI, reference nutrient intake; TUL, tolerable upper intake level.
[a]7–9 years.
[b]10–14 years.
[c]Up to the age of 18 years.
[d]19–50 years.

Dietary intake

In the UK, the average adult daily diet provides: for men, 83.4 mg; for women, 81.0 mg.

Action

Vitamin C has a wide variety of functions: the formation of collagen and other intercellular matrices in bones, teeth and capillaries; metabolism of phenylalanine, tyrosine, folic acid and histamine; conversion of ferric to ferrous iron to facilitate absorption; wound healing; immune response; an antioxidant.

Dietary sources

The richest food source is acerola cherry. Other good sources are green and red peppers, broccoli, spinach, potatoes, tomatoes, strawberries, kiwi, orange, grapefruit and other citrus fruit.

Possible uses[1,2]

Health effect or disease risk	Strength of evidence
Treats the common cold	I
Prevents the common cold	I
Enhanced immunity	I
Enhanced exercise performance	I
Protects against cataract	P
Protects against cancer	I
Protects against CVD	P
Wound healing	PR
Improves periodontal disease	P

I, insufficient; P, possible; PR, probable.

Precautions/contraindications

Caution in: diabetes mellitus (because of possible interference with glucose determinations); glucose-6-phosphate dehydrogenase (G6PD) deficiency (risk of haemolytic anaemia); haemochromatosis; sickle cell anaemia (risk of precipitating a crisis); sideroblastic anaemia; and thalassaemia. Prolonged administration of large doses (> 1 g daily) of vitamin C in pregnancy may result in increased requirements and scurvy in the neonate.

Adverse effects

Doses > 1g daily are associated with osmotic diarrhoea (caused by large amounts of unabsorbed ascorbic acid in the intestine), gastric discomfort and mild increase in urination. Doses ≥ 2 g are associated with an increased risk of oxalate stones. Prolonged use of chewable vitamin C products may cause dental erosion and increased incidence of caries.

Interactions

Drugs

Aspirin: prolonged administration may reduce blood levels of ascorbic acid.
Anticoagulants: occasional reports that vitamin C reduces the activity of warfarin.
Anticonvulsants: administration of barbiturates or primidone may increase urinary excretion of ascorbic acid.

Desferrioxamine: iron excretion induced by desferrioxamine is enhanced by administration of vitamin C.
Disulfiram: prolonged administration of large doses (> 1 g daily) of vitamin C may interfere with the alcohol–disulfiram reaction.
Mexiletine: large doses (> 1 g daily) of ascorbic acid may accelerate excretion of mexiletine.
Oral contraceptives (containing oestrogens): may reduce blood levels of ascorbic acid; large doses (> 1 g) of vitamin C may increase plasma oestrogen levels (possibly converting a low-dose to a high-dose oral contraceptive); possibly breakthrough bleeding associated with withdrawal of high-dose vitamin C.
Tetracyclines: prolonged administration may reduce blood levels of ascorbic acid.

Nutrients

Copper: high doses of vitamin C (> 1 g daily) may reduce copper retention.
Iron: vitamin C increases absorption of non-haem iron, but not haem iron. For maximal iron absorption from a non-meat meal, a source of vitamin C providing 50–100 mg should be ingested. Vitamin C supplements appear to have no deleterious effect on iron status in patients with iron overload. Iron administration reduces blood levels of ascorbic acid (ascorbic acid is oxidised).
Vitamin A: vitamin C may reduce the toxic effects of vitamin A.
Vitamin B_6: deficiency of vitamin C may increase urinary excretion of pyridoxine.
Vitamin B_{12}: excess vitamin C has been claimed to destroy vitamin B_{12}, but this does not appear to occur under physiological conditions.
Vitamin E: vitamin C can spare vitamin E, and vice versa.

Heavy metals

Vitamin C may reduce tissue and plasma levels of cadmium, lead, mercury, nickel and vanadium.

Dose

Vitamin C is available in the form of tablets, chewable tablets, capsules and powders. It is found in most multivitamin preparations. Dietary supplements contain between 25 and 1500 mg per daily dose.

References

1. Douglas RM, Hemila H, Chalker E, Treacy B. Vitamin C for preventing and treating the common cold. *Cochrane Database Syst Rev* 2007(3): CD000980.
2. Li Y, Schellhorn HE. New developments and novel therapeutic perspectives for vitamin C. *J Nutr* 2007; 137: 2171–2184.

Vitamin D

Description

Vitamin D is a fat-soluble vitamin. It is a group of several sterols, but the two most important are vitamin D_2 (ergocalciferol), obtained from irradiation of the provitamin ergosterol found in plants, and vitamin D_3 (cholecalciferol), produced under the skin from 7-dehydrocholesterol on exposure to ultraviolet light from the sun.

Human requirements

1 mcg Vitamin D = 40 units vitamin D.

DRVs for vitamin D

Age	UK		USA		FAO/WHO
	RNI (mcg/day)	EVM (mcg/day)	AI (mcg/day)	TUL (mcg/day)	RNI (mcg/day)
Males and females					
0–6 months	8.5		5	25	5
7–12 months	7.0		5	25	5
1–3 years	7.0		5	50	5
4–18 years	0[a]		5	50	5
19–50 years	0[a]	25	5	50	5
51–65 years	–	–	–	–	10
65+ years	10	25	–	–	2.5
51–70+ years	–	25	10	50	–
>65 years	–	–	–	–	15
>70 years	–	–	15	50	–
Pregnancy and lactation	10	–	5	50	10

EU RDA = 5 mcg.
AI, adequate intake; EU RDA, European Union recommended daily allowance; EVM, likely safe daily intake from supplements alone; RNI, reference nutrient intake; TUL, tolerable upper intake level.
[a]If skin is exposed to adequate sunlight.

Dietary intake

In the UK, the average adult daily diet provides: for men, 3.7 mcg, for women, 2.8 mcg.

Action

Vitamin D is a vitamin and a prohormone. It is necessary for the formation of the skeleton and mineral homeostasis, initiates production of calcium-binding protein that promotes absorption of calcium, and helps to regulate plasma calcium by increasing bone resorption and by stimulating reabsorption of calcium by the kidney.

Dietary sources

Major sources are fish liver oil and foods fortified with vitamin D; smaller amounts are found in liver, egg yolk, sardines and salmon.

Possible uses[1-4]

Health effect or disease risk	Strength of evidence
Prevention and treatment of deficiency	C
Necessary for bone health	C
Necessary for calcium absorption	C
Reduces risk of osteoporosis and fracture	PR
Reduces risk of colon cancer	P
Reduces risk of CVD	I

C, convincing; I, insufficient; P, possible; PR, probable.

Vitamin D supplements are recommended in: infants who are breastfed without supplemental vitamin D or who have minimal exposure to sunlight (the Department of Health[2] advises that all the following groups should receive supplements of vitamins A and D: all children from the age of 1–5 years; breastfeeding women; older people whose exposure to sunlight may be reduced because of poor mobility; individuals with dark skins; and those with poor exposure to sunlight).

Precautions/contraindications

Hypercalcaemia and renal osteodystrophy with hyperphosphataemia (risk of metastatic calcification).

Pregnancy/breastfeeding

No problems reported with normal intakes. There is a risk of hypercalcaemic tetany in breastfed infants whose mothers take excessive doses of vitamin D.

Adverse effects

Vitamin D is potentially toxic. Excessive intake causes anorexia, nausea, calcification of soft tissues and renal damage.

Interactions

Drugs

Anticonvulsants (phenytoin, barbiturates or primidone): may reduce effect of vitamin D by accelerating its metabolism; patients on long-term anticonvulsant therapy may require vitamin D supplementation to prevent osteomalacia.
Calcitonin: effect of calcitonin may be antagonised by vitamin D.
Colestyramine, colestipol: may reduce intestinal absorption of vitamin D.
Digoxin: caution because hypercalcaemia caused by vitamin D may potentiate effects of digoxin, resulting in cardiac arrhythmias.
Liquid paraffin: may reduce intestinal absorption of vitamin D (avoid long-term administration of liquid paraffin).
Sucralfate: may reduce intestinal absorption of vitamin D.
Thiazide diuretics: may increase risk of hypercalcaemia.
Vitamin D analogues (alfacalcidol, calcitriol, dihydrotachysterol): increased risk of toxicity with vitamin D supplements.

Nutrients

Calcium: may increase risk of hypercalcaemia.

Dose

Vitamin D is available in the form of tablets and capsules, as well as in multivitamin preparations and fish oils. A suitable dose of vitamin D in most cases is 10 mcg (400 units) daily. For prevention of fracture in older people, there is evidence that a higher dose of 20 mcg (800 units) with calcium 1200 mg daily is required.

References

1. Cranney A, Horsley T, O'Donnell S *et al*. Effectiveness and safety of vitamin D in relation to bone health. *Evid Rep Technol Assess (Full Rep)* 2007(158): 1–235.

2. Holick M. Vitamin D: importance in the prevention of cancers, type 1 diabetes, heart disease, and osteoporosis. *Am J Clin Nutr* 2004; 79: 362–371.
3. Holick M. Sunlight and vitamin D for bone health and prevention of autoimmune diseases, cancers, and cardiovascular disease. *Am J Clin Nutr* 2004;80: S1678–S1688.
4. Holick M. The vitamin D epidemic and its health consequences. *J Nutr* 2005;135: S2739–S2748.

Vitamin E

Description

Vitamin E is a fat-soluble vitamin. It consists of two groups of compounds: tocopherols and tocotrienols. Alpha-tocopherol is the most active form in humans. The form in food and natural supplements is *d*-alpha-tocopherol. The synthetic form used in many food supplements and fortified foods is *d,l*-alpha-tocopherol. The natural form is twice as potent as the synthetic form.

100 IU of natural vitamin E = 66.7 mg alpha-tocopherol; 100 IU of synthetic vitamin E = 45 mg alpha-tocopherol.

Human requirements

DRVs for vitamin E

Age	UK		USA			FAO/WHO
	Safe intake (mg/day)	EVM (mg/day)	EAR (mg/day)	RDA (mg/day)	TUL (mg/day)	RNI (mg/day)
0–6 months	0.4 mg/g PUFA		–	4[a]	–	2.7
7–12 months	0.4 mg/g PUFA		–	6[a]	–	2.7
1–3 years	0.4 mg/g PUFA		5	6	200	5.0
4–8 years	–		6	7	300	5.0[e]
9–13 years	–		9	11	600	–
10–65+ years	–				–	7.5[f]/ 10.0[g]
14–70+ years	–		12	15	1000[b]	

Males 11–50+ years	>4		–	727	–	–
Females 11–50+ years	>3		–	–	–	–
Pregnancy	–		16	19	800[c]/ 1000[d]	
Lactation	–		16	19	800[c]/ 1000[d]	

EU RDA = 10 mg.
EAR, estimated average requirement; EU RDA, European Union recommended daily allowance; EVM, likely safe daily intake from supplements alone; PUFA, polyunsaturated fatty acid; RDA, recommended daily allowance; RNI, reference nutrient intake; TUL, tolerable upper intake level.
[a]Adequate intakes (AIs).
[b]14–18 years, 800 mg.
[c]Up to 18 years.
[d]19–50 years.
[e]7–9 years, 7.0 mg.
[f]Women
[g]Men.

Dietary intake

In the UK, the average adult daily diet provides 8.3 mg.

Action

Antioxidant: protects cell membranes from toxic compounds, heavy metals and free radical damage. It is important for the development and maintenance of nerve and muscle function.

Dietary sources

Wheat germ oil; soyabean, sunflower, safflower and corn oils; meats, fish, fruit and vegetables have little vitamin E

Possible uses[1-3]

Health effect or disease risk	Strength of evidence
Reduces risk of CVD	I
Prevents cancer	I

continued

(*continued*)

Improves immunity in older people	P
Prevents cataract	P
Improvement in diabetic control	I
Slows progression of neuropsychiatric disorders	P

I, insufficient; P, possible.

Precautions/contraindications

Caution in patients taking oral anticoagulants (increased bleeding tendency), in iron-deficiency anaemia (vitamin E may impair haematological response to iron) and in hyperthyroidism.

Pregnancy/breastfeeding

No problems reported at normal intakes.

Adverse effects

At high doses: fatigue, weakness, blurred vision, headache. Does >100 times the RDA may cause bleeding after surgery.

Interactions

Drugs

Anticoagulants: large doses of vitamin E may increase the anticoagulant effect.
Anticonvulsants (phenobarbital, phenytoin, carbamazepine): may reduce plasma levels of vitamin E.
Colestyramine or colestipol: may reduce intestinal absorption of vitamin E.
Digoxin: requirement for digoxin may be reduced with vitamin E (monitoring recommended).
Insulin: requirement for insulin may be reduced by vitamin E (monitoring recommended).
Liquid paraffin: may reduce intestinal absorption of vitamin E (avoid long-term use of liquid paraffin).
Oral contraceptives: may reduce plasma vitamin E levels.
Sucralfate: may reduce intestinal absorption of vitamin E.

Nutrients

Copper: large doses of copper may increase requirement for vitamin E.
Iron: large doses of iron may increase requirements for vitamin E; vitamin E may impair the haematological response in iron-deficiency anaemia.

Polyunsaturated fatty acids (PUFAs): the dietary requirement for vitamin E increases when the intake of PUFAs increases.
Vitamin A: vitamin E spares vitamin A and protects against some signs of vitamin A toxicity; very high levels of vitamin A may increase requirement of vitamin E; excessive doses of vitamin E may deplete vitamin A.
Vitamin C: vitamin C can spare vitamin E; vitamin E can spare vitamin C.
Vitamin K: large doses of vitamin E (1200 mg daily) increase the vitamin K requirement in patients taking anticoagulants.
Zinc: zinc deficiency may result in reduced plasma vitamin E levels.

Dose

Dietary supplements provide 10–1000 mg per daily dose. Doses for use as an over-the-counter supplement above the RDA have not been established to be of value.

References

1. Stocker R. Vitamin E. *Novartis Found Symp* 2007; 282: 77–87; discussion 87–92, 212–218.
2. Blumberg JB, Frei B. Why clinical trials of vitamin E and cardiovascular diseases may be fatally flawed. Commentary on 'The relationship between dose of vitamin E and suppression of oxidative stress in humans'. *Free Radic Biol Med* 2007; 43: 1374–1376.
3. Blumberg JB. An update: vitamin E supplementation and heart disease. *Nutr Clin Care* 2002; 5: 50–55.

Vitamin K

Description

Vitamin K is a fat-soluble vitamin. Compounds with vitamin K activity: vitamin K_1 (phylloquinone) found in plants; vitamin K_2 (menaquinone) formed by bacterial synthesis in the intestine; vitamins K_3–K_7, which are synthetic preparations (of which the most active is vitamin K_3 [menadione]).

Human requirements

Vitamin K can also be synthesised in the gut.

DRVs for vitamin K				
Age	UK		USA	FAO/WHO
	Safe intake (mcg/day)	EVM (mcg/day)	RDA (mcg/day)	RNI (mcg/day)
0–6 months	10		2.0[a]	5
7–12 months	10		2.5[a]	10
1–3 years	–		30[a]	15
4–6 years	–		–	20
4–8 years	–		55[a]	–
7–9 years	–		–	25
9–13 years	–		60	–
10–18 years	–		–	35–55
14–18 years	–		75	–
Males 19–70+ years	1 mcg/kg body weight	1000	120	65
Females 19–70+ years	1 mcg/kg/ body weight	1000	90	55

Pregnancy	1 mcg/kg/ body weight		90	–
Lactation	1 mcg/kg/ body weight		90	–

EVM, likely safe daily intake from supplements alone; RDA, recommended daily allowance; RNI, reference nutrient intake.
Some of the requirement for vitamin K is met by synthesis in the intestine.
[a]Adequate intakes (AI).

Action

Essential for the formation of prothrombin and other coagulation factors involved in the regulation of blood clotting; also required for synthesis of certain proteins (found in bone, plasma and kidney) that bind calcium ions and function in bone formation and respiratory enzymes.

Dietary sources

Green vegetables: spinach, kale, broccoli and cauliflower.

Possible uses[1]

Health effect or disease risk	Strength of evidence
Reduced risk of osteoporosis and fracture	P

P, possible.

Precautions/contraindications

None reported (except Interactions – see below).

Pregnancy/breastfeeding

No problems reported.

Adverse effects

Oral ingestion of natural forms of vitamin K is not associated with toxicity. A rare hypersensitivity reaction (occasionally results in death) has been reported after intravenous administration of phytomenadione (especially if rapid).

Interactions

Drugs

Antibiotics: may increase requirement for vitamin K.
Anticoagulants: anticoagulant effect reduced by vitamin K (vitamin K is present in several tube feeds); dosage adjustment of anticoagulant may be necessary, especially when vitamin K has been used to antagonise excessive effects of anticoagulants (see the *British National Formulary*).
Colestyramine or colestipol: may reduce intestinal absorption of vitamin K.
Liquid paraffin: may reduce intestinal absorption of vitamin K (avoid long-term use of liquid paraffin).
Sucralfate: may reduce intestinal absorption of vitamin K.

Nutrients

Vitamin A: under conditions of hypervitaminosis A, hypothrombinaemia may occur; it can be corrected by administering vitamin K.
Vitamin E: large doses of vitamin E (1200 mg daily) increase the vitamin K requirement in patients taking anticoagulants, but no confirmed effect in individuals not taking anticoagulants.

Dose

Vitamin K is not generally available in isolation as a supplement. It is an ingredient in some multivitamin preparations. No dose has been established.

Reference

1. Francucci CM, Rilli S, Fiscaletti P, Boscaro M. Role of vitamin K on biochemical markers, bone mineral density, and fracture risk. *J Endocrinol Invest* 2007; 30 (6 suppl): 24–28.

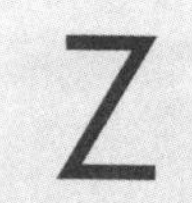

Zinc

Description

Zinc is an essential trace mineral.

Human requirements

DRVs for zinc							
Age	UK				USA		FAO/ WHO
	LNRI (mg/ day)	EAR (mg/ day)	RNI (mg/ day)	EVM (mg/ day)	RDA (mg/ day)	TUL (mg/ day)	RNI[b] (mg/ day)
0–3 months	2.6	3.3	4.0		2.0[e]	0	1.1–6.6
4–6 months	2.6	3.3	4.0		2.0[e]	0	1.1–6.6
7–12 months	3.0	3.8	5.0		3.0	5.0	2.5–8.4
1–3 years	3.0	3.8	5.0		3.0	7.0	2.4–8.3
4–6 years	4.0	5.0	6.5		–	–	2.9–9.6
4–8 years	–	–	–		5.0	12.0	–
7–10 years	4.0	5.4	7.0		–	–	3.3–11.2[c]
Males 11–14 years	5.3	7.0	9.0		–	–	5.1–17.1[d]

continued

(continued)

14–18 years	–	–	–		11.0	34.0	5.1–17.1
15–18 years	5.5	7.3	9.5		–	–	–
19–50+ years	5.5	7.3	9.5	25	11.0	40.0	–
19–65+ years	–	–	–		–	–	4.2–14.0
Females							
11–14 years	5.3	7.0	9.0		–	–	4.3–14.4[d]
14–18 years	–	–	–		9.0	34.0	4.3–14.4
15–18 years	4.0	5.5	7.0		–	–	–
19–50+ years	4.0	5.5	7.0	25	8.0	40.0	–
19–65+ years	–	–	–		–	–	3.0–9.8
Pregnancy	[a]	[a]	[a]		11.0[f]	40.0[g]	–
Lactation	–	–	–		12.0[h]	40.0[g]	–
0–4 months			+6.0		–	–	–
4+ months			+2.5		–	–	–

EU RDA = 15 mg.
EAR, estimated average requirement; EU RDA, European Union recommended daily allowance; EVM, likely safe daily intake from supplements alone; LNRI, lower reference nutrient intake; RDA, recommended daily allowance; RNI, reference nutrient intake; TUL, tolerable upper intake level.
[a]No increment.
[b]Recommended intake varies from diet of high to low zinc bioavailability.
[c]7–9 years.
[d]10–14 years.
[e]Adequate intakes (AIs).
[f]Aged < 18 years, 13 mg daily.
[g]Aged < 18 years, 34 mg daily.
[h]Aged < 18 years, 14 mg daily.

Dietary intake

In the UK, the average adult daily diet provides: for men, 10.2 mg; for women, 7.4 mg.

Action

A cofactor in more than 100 different enzymes, zinc is involved in: carbohydrate, protein and energy metabolism; nucleic acid synthesis; acid–base balance; carbon dioxide transport; metabolism of vitamin A and collagen; thyroid function; maintenance of taste acuity; development of reproductive organs; sperm production; fetal development and growth of children; and disposal of free radicals.

Dietary sources

Oysters, red meat, poultry, liver and kidney, shellfish and seafood, cereals, whole grains, fortified breakfast cereals, legumes and nuts.

Possible uses[1-4]

Health effect or disease risk	Strength of evidence
Treatment of cold	I
Improves age-related macular degeneration	P
Treats acne	I
Wound healing (in people with low zinc)	PR
Male fertility	I
Benign prostatic hyperplasia	I
Improves exercise performance	I
Improves immunity in older people	I

I, insufficient; P, possible; PR, probable.

Precautions/contraindications

Caution in prolonged use as a single supplement.

Pregnancy/breastfeeding

See precautions.

Adverse effects

Prolonged intake can result in: copper deficiency; reduced iron status; depressed levels of white blood cells; increased LDL- and decreased HDL-cholesterol.

Interactions

Drugs

Ciprofloxacin: reduced absorption of ciprofloxacin.
Oral contraceptives: may reduce plasma zinc levels.
Penicillamine: reduced absorption of penicillamine.
Tetracyclines: reduced absorption of zinc and vice versa.

Nutrients

Copper: large doses of zinc may reduce absorption of copper.
Folic acid: may reduce zinc absorption (raises concern about pregnant women who are advised to take folic acid to reduce the risk of birth defects).
Iron: reduces absorption of oral iron and vice versa (raises concern about pregnant women who are often given iron; this may reduce zinc status and increase the risk of intrauterine growth retardation and congenital abnormalities in the fetus).

Dose

The dose beyond the RDA is not established. Dietary supplements contain 5–50 mg (elemental zinc) per daily dose.

The zinc content of some commonly used zinc salts is as follows: zinc amino acid chelate (100 mg/g); zinc gluconate (130 mg/g); zinc orotate (170 mg/g); zinc sulphate (227 mg/g).

References

1. Caruso TJ, Prober CG, Gwaltney JM, Jr. Treatment of naturally acquired common colds with zinc: a structured review. *Clin Infect Dis* 2007;45: 569–574.
2. Vasto S, Mocchegiani E, Malavolta M *et al*. Zinc and inflammatory/immune response in aging. *Ann N Y Acad Sci* 2007;1100: 111–122.
3. Lansdown AB, Mirastschijski U, Stubbs N, Scanlon E, Agren MS. Zinc in wound healing: theoretical, experimental, and clinical aspects. *Wound Repair Regen* 2007;15(1): 2–16.
4. Costello LC, Franklin RB, Feng P, Tan M, Bagasra O. Zinc and prostate cancer: a critical scientific, medical, and public interest issue (United States). *Cancer Causes Control* 2005;16: 901–915.

Appendix 1

Guidance on safe upper levels of vitamins and minerals

Vitamin/mineral	EU RDA	EVM UK	TUL USA	SCF EU
Vitamin A (retinol equivalent mcg)	800	1500[1]	3000	3600
Vitamin B_1 (thiamine) mg	1.4	100[1]	–	
Vitamin B_2 (riboflavin) mg	1.6	100[1]	–	–
Vitamin B_6 (pyridoxine) mg	2	10[2]	100	25
Vitamin B_{12} (cobalamin) mcg	1	1000[1]	–	–
Vitamin C (ascorbic acid) mg	60	1000[1]	2000	–
Vitamin D (cholecalciferol) mcg	5	25[1]	50	50
Vitamin E (tocopherol) mg	10	727[2]	1000	300
Niacin mg	18		30	
Nicotinamide mg	–	500[1]		900
Nicotinic acid mg	–	17[1]		10
Biotin mcg	150	970[1]	–	–
Folic acid mcg	200	1000[1]	1000	1000
Pantothenic acid mg	6	200[1]	–	–
Calcium mg	800	1500[1]	2500	2500
Iodine mcg	150	500[1]	1100	600
Iron mg	14	17[1]	45	
Magnesium mg	300	400[1]	350	250
Phosphorus mg	800	250[1]	4000	

continued

(continued)

Zinc mg	15	25[2]	40	25
Vitamin K mg	–	1[1]	–	–
Beta-carotene mg		7[2]	–	20
Chromium mcg	–	–	–	
Copper mg	5[2]	10	5	
Manganese mg		4[1]	11	–
Molybdenum mcg		–	2000	600
Selenium mcg	–	200[2]	400	300
Boron mg	–	5.9[2]	20	
Nickel mg	–		1	
Vanadium mg	–		1.8	–

EU RDA: the Recommended Daily Allowance considered sufficient to prevent deficiency in most individuals in the population.
EVM: draft figures (2002) produced by the Food Standards Agency (FSA) Expert Vitamin and Mineral (EVM) group.
[1]Likely safe total daily intake from supplements alone.
[2]Safe upper level from supplements alone.
TUL: Tolerable Upper Intake Levels defined by the Food and Nutrition Board of the US National Academy of Sciences as the highest total level of a nutrient (diet plus supplements) that could be consumed safely on a daily basis, which is unlikely to cause adverse health effects to almost all individuals in the general population. As intakes rise above the TUL, the risk of adverse effects increases. The TUL describes long-term intakes, so an isolated dose above the TUL need not necessarily cause adverse effects. The TUL defines safety limits and is not a recommended intake for most people most of the time.
SCF: Tolerable Upper Intake Levels defined by the European Commission's Scientific Committee on Food (SCF) as the maximum level of chronic daily intake of a nutrient (from all sources) judged to be unlikely to pose a risk of adverse effects to humans. http://ec.europa.eu/comm./food/fs/sc/scf/out80_en.html
Note: dashes (–) indicate that the nutrient has been considered but no level set. Where the column is blank, the nutrient has not been considered.

Appendix 2

Drug and supplement interactions

Drug	Food/ nutrient	Effect	Intervention
Drugs acting on the gastrointestinal system			
Antacids	Iron	Aluminium-, magnesium- and calcium-containing antacids and sodium bicarbonate reduce absorption of iron	Separate administration of antacids and iron by at least 2 h
Sulfasalazine	Folic acid	Sulfasalazine can reduce absorption of folic acid	Monitor and give a supplement if necessary
Stimulant laxatives	Potassium	Prolonged use of stimulant laxatives can precipitate hypokalaemia	Avoid prolonged use of laxatives
Liquid paraffin	Fat-soluble vitamins	Liquid paraffin reduces absorption of vitamins A, D, E and K	Avoid prolonged use of liquid paraffin
Drugs acting in the treatment of diseases of the cardiovascular system			
Thiazide diuretics	Calcium/ vitamin D	Excessive serum calcium levels can develop in patients given thiazides with supplements of calcium and/or vitamin D	Concurrent use of thiazides with calcium and/or vitamin D need not be avoided but serum calcium levels should be monitored
ACE inhibitors	Potassium	Concurrent use of ACE inhibitors with potassium may induce severe hyperkalaemia	Avoid

continued

(continued)

Potassium-sparing diuretics	Potassium	Concurrent use of potassium-sparing diuretics and either potassium supplements or potassium-containing salt substitutes may induce severe hyperkalaemia	Avoid concurrent use of potassium-sparing diuretics and potassium supplements unless potassium levels are monitored; warn patients about risks of salt substitutes
Calcium-channel blockers	Calcium	Therapeutic effects of verapamil can be antagonised by calcium	Calcium supplements should be used with caution in patients taking verapamil
Hydralazine	Vitamin B_6	Long-term administration of hydralazine may lead to pyridoxine deficiency	Vitamin B_6 supplement may be needed if symptoms of peripheral neuritis develop
Anticoagulants	Vitamin E	Effects of warfarin may be increased by large doses of vitamin E	Avoid high-dose vitamin E supplements
	Vitamin K	Effects of anticoagulants can be reduced or abolished by large intakes of vitamin K	Avoid excessive intake of vitamin K (e.g. check labels of enteral feeds)
	Bromelain	Effects of anticoagulants may be increased by these supplements	Care with these supplements in people taking anticoagulants, aspirin and anti-platelet drugs. Avoid if possible, otherwise monitor carefully
	Chondroitin		
	Fish oils		
	Garlic		
	Ginkgo biloba		

	Ginseng		
	Grape seed extract		
	Green tea		
	S-Adenosyl methionine		
Colestyramine	Fat-soluble vitamins	Prolonged use of these drugs may result in deficiency of fat-soluble vitamins	Supplements of vitamins A, D, E and K may be needed if these drugs are administered for prolonged periods
Colestipol			
Drugs acting on the central nervous system			
Phenothiazines	Evening primrose oil	Evening primrose oil supplements may increase the risk of epileptic side-effects	Avoid evening primrose oil supplements
Monoamine oxidase inhibitors	Brewers' yeast	Brewers' yeast may provoke a hypertensive crisis	Avoid brewers' yeast supplements
Anti-epileptics*	Folic acid	Anti-epileptics may cause folate deficiency, but use of folic acid supplements may lead to a fall in serum anticonvulsant levels and reduced seizure control	Folic acid supplements should be given only to those folate-deficient patients on anti-epileptics who can be monitored
	Vitamin B_6	Large doses of vitamin B_6 may reduce serum levels of phenytoin and phenobarbitone	Avoid large doses of vitamin B_6 from supplements (>10 mg daily)
	Vitamin D	Anti-epileptics may disturb metabolism of vitamin D leading to osteomalacia	Susceptible individuals should take 10 mcg vitamin D daily

continued

(*continued*)

	Vitamin K	Anti-epileptics have been associated with fetal haemorrhage. This is because the drug crosses the placenta and decreases vitamin K status, resulting in bleeding in the infant	Vitamin K should be provided to the newborn infant
Levodopa	Iron	Iron reduces the absorption of levodopa	Separate doses of iron and levodopa by at least 2 h
	Vitamin B_6	Effects of levodopa are reduced or abolished by vitamin B_6 supplements (>5 mg daily), but dietary vitamin B_6 has no effect	Avoid all supplements containing any vitamin B_6. Suggest co-careldopa or co-beneldopa as an alternative to levodopa
Drugs used in the treatment of infections			
Tetracyclines	Iron	Absorption of tetracyclines is reduced by iron and vice versa	Separate doses of iron and tetracyclines by at least 2 h
	Calcium/ magnesium/ zinc	Absorption of tetracyclines may be reduced by mineral supplements and vice versa	Separate doses of mineral supplements and tetracyclines by at least 2 h
Trimethoprim	Folic acid	Folate deficiency in susceptible individuals	Folic acid supplement may be needed if drug used for prolonged periods
4-Quinolones	Iron/zinc	Absorption of 4-quinolones may be reduced by mineral supplements and vice versa	Separate doses of mineral supplements and 4-quinolones by at least 2 h

Cycloserine	Folic acid	Folate deficiency in susceptible individuals	Monitor folate status and give supplement if necessary
Isoniazid	Vitamin B_6	Long-term administration of isoniazid may lead to pyridoxine deficiency	Vitamin B_6 supplement may be needed if symptoms of peripheral neuritis develop
Rifampicin	Vitamin D	Rifampicin may disturb metabolism of vitamin D leading to osteomalacia in susceptible individuals	Monitor serum vitamin D levels
Drugs used in the treatment of disorders of the endocrine system			
Oral hypoglycaemics and insulin	Aloe vera	These supplements could theoretically potentiate the effects of oral hypoglycaemics and insulin	Care in people on medication for diabetes
	Alpha-lipoic acid		
	Chromium		
	Glucosamine	Glucosamine might reduce the effects of oral hypoglycaemics and insulin	Care in people on medication for diabetes
Oestrogens (including HRT and oral contraceptives)	Vitamin C	Concurrent administration of oestrogens and large doses of vitamin C (1 g daily) increases serum levels of oestrogens	Avoid high-dose vitamin C supplements
	DHEA	May potentiate hormonal effects	Care in people using HRT
	Isoflavones	May potentiate hormonal effects	Care in people using HRT

continued

(continued)

Bisphosphonates	Calcium	May lead to reduced absorption of bisphosphonate	Take 2 h apart
Thyroid medication	Kelp/iodine	May lead to poor control of thyroid condition	Avoid without a doctor's advice.
Drugs used in the treatment of musculo-skeletal and joint diseases			
Penicillamine	Iron/zinc	Absorption of penicillamine reduced by mineral supplements and vice versa	Separate doses of mineral supplements and penicillamine by at least 2 h

*This interaction applies to the older anti-epileptic drugs (e.g. phenytoin, primidine, phenobarbitone, valproate and carbamazepine). There is little information on newer anti-epileptic drugs except with the possibility of lamotrigine, which may have anti-epileptic properties. (Gilman JT. Lamotrigine: an antiepileptic agent for the treatment of partial seizures. *Ann Pharmacother* 1995; 29: 144–151.)

Appendix 3

Additional resources

Government web sites related to dietary supplements

United Kingdom

UK Food Standards Agency Expert Group on Vitamins and Minerals (EVM): A group of independent experts established to consider the safety of vitamins and minerals sold under food law. Produced a report, *Safe Upper Levels for Vitamins and Minerals*, in May 2003.
http://www.food.gov.uk

Medicines and Healthcare products Regulatory Agency (MHRA): The UK body that licenses medicines. Provides information on legislation relating to herbals and supplements.
http://www.mhra.gov.uk

Europe

European Union Food Safety web site: Gives details of all EU regulation on food supplements.
http://www.europa.eu/pol/food/index_en.htm

European Food Safety Authority (EFSA): http://ec.europa.eu/comm./food/efsa/efsa_admin_en.htm

USA

US Food and Drug Administration (FDA): FDA Center for Food Safety and Applied Nutrition
http://vm.cfsan.fda.gov/list.html

FDA press releases and fact sheets: http://vm.cfsan.fda.gov/~lrd/press.html

FDA what's new: http://vm.cfsan.fda.gov/~news/whatsnew.html

Announcements about dietary supplements: Includes details of adverse effects reported to the FDA about individual supplements.
http://vm.cfsan.fda.gov/~dms/supplmnt.html

Overview and history of FDA and the Center for Food Safety and Applied Nutrition: http://vm.cfsan.fda.gov/~lrd/fdahist.html

National Institutes of Health Office of Dietary Supplements: http://dietary-supplements.info.nih.gov

Associations representing industry

Association of the European Self-Medication Industry (AESGP): European trade association representing the over-the-counter healthcare products industry.

http://www.aesgp.be

Council for Responsible Nutrition (CRN): Provides member companies with legislative guidance, regulatory interpretation, scientific information on supplement benefits and safety issues and communications expertise.

UK web site: http://www.crn-uk.org
US web site: http://www.crnusa.org

Health Food Manufacturers' Association (HFMA): A trade association that acts as a voice for the industry; covers food supplements, health foods, herbal remedies, etc.

http://www.hfma.co.uk

International Alliance of Dietary/Food Supplement Associations (IADSA): Aims to facilitate a sound legislative and political environment to build growth in the international market for dietary supplements based on scientific principles.

http://www.iadsa.org

Proprietary Association of Great Britain (PAGB): UK trade association representing the consumer healthcare industry.

http://www.pagb.co.uk

Journals and newsletters

American Journal of Clinical Nutrition: Official journal of the American Society for Clinical Nutrition. Published monthly.

http://www.ajcn.org

Focus on Alternative and Complementary Therapies (FACT): Provides summaries and commentaries on various aspects of complementary medicine, including vitamins, minerals and supplements. Published quarterly.

http://www.pharmpress.com

Journal of Dietary Supplements: A peer-reviewed academic publication, providing the latest information on food supplements. Published quarterly.
The Haworth Press Inc.
http://www.haworthpressinc.com
Tel: +1 800 342 9678

Medicinal Foods News: An online magazine devoted to medical and functional foods.
http://www.medicinalfoodnews.com

On-line research information and comment

Arbor Nutrition Guide: Provides regular updates on nutritional issues, including those with relevance to supplements.
http://arborcom.com
(for subscriptions, see http://www.nutritionupdates.org/sub/sub01.php?item=3)

International bibliographic information on dietary supplements (IBIDS): The aim of this database is to help health professionals, researchers and the general public find scientific literature on dietary supplements.
http://ods.od/nih.gov/Health_Information/IBIDS.aspx

Medline: The US National Library of Medicine's bibliographic database providing extensive coverage of medicine and healthcare from approximately 3900 current biomedical journals, published in about 70 countries.
http://www.ncbi.nlm.nih.gov/pubmed

Medline Dietary Supplements: http://www.nlm.nih.gov/medlineplus/dietarysupplements.html

Medline Vitamins: http://www.nlm.nih.gov/medlineplus/vitamins.html

Other information

Consumer Lab: Tests the content of diet supplements in the USA and provides reports on its work.
http://consumerlab.com

Health Supplement Information Service (HSIS): Developed by the Proprietary Association of Great Britain (PAGB) to present the facts about health supplements in a straightforward way. Aims to eliminate confusion and provide reliable data about individual nutrients and supplements.
http://www.hsis.org

Eurreca: A network of scientists, nutrition societies, consumer organisations, small and medium sized enterprises and wider stakeholders funded by the European Commission (EC) to work together to address the problem of national variations in micronutrient recommendations.
http://www.eurreca.org

Quackwatch: A non-profit organisation with the aim of debunking health-related frauds, myths, fads and fallacies. There are sections on dietary supplements.
http://www.quackwatch.com/index.html

Index

Page references in bold refer to tables

ACE inhibitors 178, 257
acne 19, 26, 253
adaptogen 99
Adequate Daily Dietary Intakes viii
age-related macular degeneration *see* macular degeneration, age-related
ageing *see* anti-ageing
AIDS *see* HIV/AIDS
alcohol interactions
- calcium 34
- magnesium 138
- pantothenic acid 167
- riboflavin 197
- thiamine 217
- vitamin B_6 230
- vitamin B_{12} 234

alcoholic liver disease 201
alcoholism 217
allergic rhinitis 145, 211
- *see also* hay fever

allergies 13
allicin 93
aloe vera 1, 261
alopecia areata 19
alpha-carotene 40
alpha-linolenic acid 78, 82
alpha-lipoic acid 4, 7, 261
alpha-tocopherol 244
altitude sickness 96
Alzheimer's disease
- prevention 79, 83, 210, 211
- reducing deterioration 38, 1
- sleep enhancement 142
- symptomatic improvement 96, 134, 172
- thiamine 217

American Journal of Clinical Nutrition 264
amino acids, branched-chain (BCAAs) 24
aminoglycosides 234
aminosalicylates 234
amyotrophic lateral sclerosis 24, 161
analgesia 170
Angelica sinensis (dong quai) 70
angina 38, 55
anorexia 24
antacids 34, 52, 126, 257
anti-ageing
- chlorella 44
- dehydroepiandrosterone 67
- guarana 112
- royal jelly 198
- spirulina 211
- superoxide dismutase 213

anti-diabetic drugs 185
anti-epileptic drug interactions *see* anticonvulsant interactions
anti-platelet drugs 71
antibiotic-associated diarrhoea 181
antibiotics 29, 234, 249, 260
anticoagulant interactions 258
- chondroitin 50
- dong quai 71
- fish oil 80
- vitamin A 226
- vitamin C 238
- vitamin E 246
- vitamin K 250

anticonvulsant interactions 259

biotin 20
calcium 34
carnitine 38
folic acid 88
vitamin C 238
vitamin D 242
vitamin E 246
antidepressants 118
antioxidants 7
sources 4, 40, 105, 109, 245
see also oxidative stress
antiretroviral therapy 196
antithyroid drugs 123
anxiety 113, 117
appetite suppression 112, 137
Arbor Nutrition Guide 265
arginine 10
arthritis
antioxidants 8
bromelain 28
copper 61
fish oil 78
flaxseed oil 82
green tea extract 110
see also osteoarthritis; rheumatoid arthritis
ascorbic acid *see* vitamin C
aspirin 52, 185, 238
Association of the European Self-Medication Industry (AESGP) 264
astaxanthin 40
asthma
antioxidants 8
evening primrose oil 74
fish oil 79
green-lipped mussel 107
green tea extract 110
selenium 205
vitamin B_6 230
athletes
muscle/fat-free mass 52
recovery/free radical stress 26
stamina and endurance 112
see also ergogenic aids; exercise performance
attention 22
attention deficit hyperactivity disorder 79, 142, 170
autism 230
autoimmune disease 190
barbiturates 197, 242
bee pollen 13
behavioural problems, childhood 79
benign prostatic hyperplasia (BPH) 13, 186, 187, 253
beta-carotene 40
action 7, 40
adverse effects 9
bioavailability 41
safe upper levels 256
betaine 16
betaine hydrochloride 16
biotin 18
deficiency 19
dietary reference values **18**
safe upper levels 255
biotinidase deficiency 19
bipolar disorder 142
bisphosphonates 34, 126, 262
blood pressure lowering
garlic 82
ginseng 100
magnesium 137
potassium 177
pycnogenol 170
see also hypertension
bone
formation 179
health 179, 179, 137, 241
metabolism 58
boron 21, 256
bowel function 44
branched-chain amino acids (BCAAs) 24
breast cancer
carotenoids 40
coenzyme Q10 55
evening primrose oil 74
folic acid 87
isoflavones 129
breastfed infants 241
brewers' yeast 26, 259
bromelain 28, 258
bronchitis, chronic 153
bruising 29

burning mouth syndrome 5
burns 2
cachexia 24
cadmium 239
caffeine 64, 112
calcitonin 242
calcium 31
  absorption 241
  dietary reference values **31**
  drug interactions 257, 258, 260, 262
  nutrient interactions 127, 242
  prevention of loss 21
  safe upper levels 255
calcium-channel blockers 258
cancer
  antioxidants 8, 40, 204
  calcium 33
  carnitine 38
  conjugated linoleic acid 58
  dehydroepiandrosterone 68
  fish oil 79
  flaxseed oil 82
  folic acid 87
  garlic 94
  ginseng 100
  green tea extract 109
  melatonin 142
  phytosterols 174
  prebiotics 179
  probiotics 181
  quercetin 190
  shark cartilage 207
  superoxide dismutase 213
  vitamins 150, 226, 238, 245
  see also specific types of cancer
Candida infections 19
capillary resistance, poor 105
carbamazepine 20, 185, 246
carbenoxolone 178
carbohydrate cravings 52
carboplatin 22
cardiac glycosides 34
cardiovascular disease (CVD)
  antioxidants 8
  arginine 10
  betaine 16
  carnitine 38
  carotenoids 41
  choline 47
  coenzyme Q10 54
  dong quai 70
  fish oils 78
  flaxseed oil 82
  folic acid 87
  multivitamins 150
  phytosterols 174
  pycnogenol 170
  quercetin 190
  resveratrol 193
  selenium 204
  silicon 209
  superoxide dismutase 213
  vitamin B_6 230
  vitamin B_{12} 233
  vitamin C 238
  vitamin D 241
  vitamin E 245
carnitine 37
carotenoids 40, 44, 224
carpal tunnel syndrome 230
cataract
  antioxidants 8
  carotenoids 41
  multivitamins 150
  quercetin 190
  vitamin C 238
  vitamin E 246
cervical cancer 40, 87
chemotherapy tolerance 44
children
  acute diarrhoea 181
  behavioural problems 181
  see also attention deficit hyperactivity disorder
chitosan 42
chloramphenicol 234
chlorella 44
cholecalciferol 240, 255
cholesterol lowering
  brewers' yeast 26
  chitosan 42
  chromium 52
  copper 61
  flaxseed oil 82

gamma-oryzanol 91
garlic 94
green tea extract 109
isoflavones 128
lecithin 134
nicotinic acid 157
octacosanol 161
phytosterols 174
probiotics 181
psyllium 184, 185
pumpkin seeds 186
vanadium 222
see also lipid profile improvements
choline 46
chondroitin 49, 258
chromium 51
interactions 52, 261
safe upper levels 256
sources 26, 51
chronic fatigue syndrome 38, 142
chronic obstructive pulmonary disease (COPD) 153
ciclosporin 178
ciprofloxacin 254
circulation 94
Clarinol 58
claudication, intermittent 161
see also peripheral vascular disease
Clostridium difficile 26
clozapine 205
co-careldopa 126
cobalamin *see* vitamin B_{12}
coenzyme A 166
coenzyme Q10 7, 54
cognitive function
boron 22
fish oils 79
green tea extract 110
isoflavones 129
lecithin 134
multivitamins 150
vitamin B_6 230
see also dementia; memory enhancement
colchicine 226
cold, common 238, 253
colestipol 226, 242, 246, 250, 259
colestyramine 259
folic acid interaction 88
vitamin A interaction 226
vitamin B_{12} interaction 234
vitamin D interaction 242
vitamin E interaction 246
vitamin K interaction 250
colorectal cancer 33, 40, 87, 129, 241
congestive heart failure *see* heart failure
conjugated linoleic acid (CLA) 57
constipation 2, 14, 112, 184, 185
Consumer Lab 265
copper 60
action 7, 61
dietary reference values **60**
interactions 127, 239, 246, 254
safe upper levels 254
sources 26
coronary heart disease (CHD) 49, 77, 99, 137
see also heart disease
corticosteroids 34, 178
Council for Responsible Nutrition (CRN) 264
creatine 63
Crohn's disease 79, 182
cryptoxanthin 40
cycloserine 230, 261
cystic fibrosis 227
daidzein 128
deep vein thrombosis, prevention 170
dehydroepiandrosterone (DHEA) 67, 261
dementia 5, 79, 233
see also Alzheimer's disease; cognitive function
dental caries 84
depression
chromium 52
dehydroepiandrosterone 68
fish oils 79

folic acid 87
ginkgo biloba 96
5-hydroxytryptophan 117
phosphatidylserine 172
S-adenosyl methionine 201
desferrioxamine 239
diabetes mellitus
aloe vera 2
alpha-lipoic acid 4
biotin (improved control) 19
chromium 52
fish oils 79
folic acid 89
ginseng 100
magnesium 137
psyllium 184, 185
pumpkin seeds 186
pycnogenol 170
vitamin E 246
see also glucose
diabetic neuropathy 38, 74, 230, 234
diarrhoea 14, 26, 29, 181, 184
dietary intake ix
Dietary Reference Values (DRVs) viii
digestive function 44
digoxin 100, 185, 242, 246
disulfiram 239
diuretics 34, 138, 178, 257
docosahexaenoic acid (DHA) 77, 82
dong quai 70
drug and supplement interactions 257
dry eye syndrome 74
dry mouth 16
eczema 73, 74, 82
eicosapentaenoic acid (EPA) 77, 82
elderly *see* older people
eosinophilic myalgia syndrome (EMS) 117
erectile dysfunction 10
ergocalciferol 240
ergogenic aids 10, 63, 222
Estimated Average Requirement (EAR) viii
European Union
Recommended Dietary Allowances (RDAs) viii
web sites 263
evening primrose oil 74, 259
evidence, strength of ix
exercise performance
antioxidants 8
bee pollen 13
branched-chain amino acids 24
brewers' yeast 26
carnitine 38
choline 47
coenzyme Q10 55
creatine 63
gamma-oryzanol 91
ginseng 99
magnesium 137
vitamin C 238
zinc 253
see also athletes; ergogenic aids
fat
absorption 42
body 52, 57
fatigue 38
fibromyalgia 44, 117, 201
fish oil 77, 258
flavonoids 7, 105
flaxseed oil 82
fluoride 35, 84
Focus on Alternative and Complementary Therapies (FACT) 264
folic acid 86
dietary reference values **86**
drug interactions 88, 257, 259, 260, 261
nutrient interactions 88, 235, 254
safe upper levels 255
food allergy 182
Food and Drug Administration (FDA) 263
Food Standards Agency Expert Group on Vitamins and Minerals (EVM) 263
fracture prevention 33, 84, 241, 242, 249
free radicals 7

see also oxidative stress
fructo-oligosaccharides 179
furosemide 217
gamma-linolenic acid (GLA) 73
gamma-oryzanol 91
garlic 93, 258
genistein 128
ginkgo biloba 96, 258
ginseng 99, 259
glaucoma 5, 96, 143
glucosamine 102, 261
glucose
blood levels 26, 42, 100, 211, 222
metabolism 10
see also diabetes mellitus
glucose tolerance factor (GTF) 26, 51
glutathione (GSH) 7, 153, 201
glycetin 128
glycosaminoglycans 49, 207
goitre 123
grape seed extract 105, 259
green-lipped mussel 107
green tea extract 109, 259
guarana 112
H_2-receptor antagonists 234
haemorrhoids 29
hair
condition 45
loss 74
hand–eye coordination 22
hay fever (seasonal allergic rhinitis) 14, 105
see also allergic rhinitis
headache 117, 143
Health Food Manufacturers' Association (HFMA) 264
Health Supplement Information Service (HSIS) 265
hearing loss, age-related 4
heart disease 73, 77, 109
see also coronary heart disease
heart failure (congestive heart failure; CHF) 38, 55, 64, 100
heavy metals 239
Helicobacter pylori 181
histamine H_2-receptor antagonists 234
HIV/AIDS 4, 37, 67, 153
homocysteine 16, 47, 145, 235
homocystinuria 16
hormone replacement therapy (HRT) 261
see also oestrogens
hydralazine 230, 258
hydroxycitric acid (HCA) 115
5-hydroxytryptophan (5HTP) 117
hyperkalaemia 117
hypertension
alpha-lipoic acid 4
calcium 33
chlorella 44
coenzyme Q10 54
melatonin 142
silicon 209
see also blood pressure lowering
immune function, enhancement
arginine 11
bee pollen 14
chlorella 44
conjugated linoleic acid 57
dehydroepiandrosterone 67
ginseng 99
guarana 112
prebiotics 179
probiotics 181
selenium 204
vitamin C 238
vitamin E 245
zinc 253
infants, breastfed 241
infections 2, 149, 179
infertility, male 38, 253
inflammatory bowel disease 79, 103
see also Crohn's disease; ulcerative colitis
influenza 153
insect repellant 217
insomnia 117, 142
insulin
interactions 53, 246, 261
resistance 57, 109
sensitivity 67, 140, 221
intermittent claudication 161

see also peripheral vascular disease
International Alliance of Dietary/ Food Supplement Associations (IADSA) 264
International Aloe Science Council (IASC) 3
International bibliographic information of dietary supplements (IBIDS) 265
inulin 179
iodine 122, 131
dietary reference values **121**
interactions 123, 257
safe upper levels 255
iron 124
deficiency 126
dietary reference values **124**
drug interactions 257, 260, 260, 260, 262
nutrient interactions 35, 62, 197, 227, 239, 246, 254
safe upper levels 255
sources 26, 44, 211
irritable bowel syndrome (IBS)
aloe vera 2
melatonin 143
prebiotics 179
probiotics 182
psyllium 184, 185
pumpkin seeds 186
isoflavones 128, 261
isoniazid 230, 261
ispaghula (psyllium) 184
jet lag 142, 184
Joint Health Claims Initiative (JHCI) 266
Journal of Dietary Supplements 265
kelp 131, 262
kidney stones 186
lactic acidosis 196
lactobacilli 181
lactose intolerance 181
lamotrigine 262
laxatives 34, 178, 257
lead 239
lecithin 46, 133
levodopa 126, 231, 260
linoleic acid 186
conjugated (CLA) 57
linolenic acid 186
alpha 78, 82
gamma (GLA) 73
lipid-lowering drugs 157, 226
see also colestipol; colestyramine; statins
lipid peroxidation 47
lipid profile improvements
carnitine 37
conjugated linoleic acid 58
grape seed extract 105
hydroxycitric acid 115
prebiotics 179
spirulina 211
see also cholesterol lowering
lipoic acid *see* alpha-lipoic acid
liquid paraffin 226, 242, 246, 249, 257
lithium 185
loop diuretics 34, 138, 177
Lower Reference Nutrient Intake (LRNI) viii
lung cancer 40, 153
lupus 68, 82
lupus erythematosus, systemic 79
lutein 7, 40
lycopene 7, 40
macular degeneration, age-related
antioxidants 8
ginkgo biloba 97
melatonin 143
multivitamins 150
zinc 253
magnesium 135
dietary reference values **135**
interactions 22, 138, 260
safe upper levels 255
manganese 139
dietary reference values **139**
interactions 127, 141
safe upper levels 255
mastalgia 75
Medicinal Foods News 265
Medicines and Healthcare products Regulatory Agency (MHRA) 263

Medline 265
melatonin 142
memory enhancement
bee pollen 13
boron 22
choline 46
dehydroepiandrosterone 78
ginkgo biloba 96
lecithin 133
see also cognitive function; dementia
menadione 248
menaquinone 248
menopausal symptoms 270,100, 110, 129
menstrual pain 28, 33
mental alertness 113
mental performance 8, 99
mercury 239
metformin 234
methotrexate 88, 89
methyldopa 126, 234
methylsulfonylmethane (MSM) 145
mexiletine 239
migraine
alpha-lipoic acid 5
coenzyme Q10 55
guarana 113
magnesium 137
riboflavin 196
minerals
absorption 179
psyllium interactions 185
safe upper levels 255
molybdenum 147
dietary reference values **138**
safe upper levels 256
monoamine oxidase inhibitors (MAOIs) 26, 118, 204, 259
mood disorders 79
see also bipolar disorder; depression
mood enhancement 205
mountain sickness 96
mouth ulcers 2, 216, 234
multiple sclerosis 97, 233
multivitamins 149
muscle strength 64
musculoskeletal injuries 28
N-acetylcysteine (NAC) 153
nails 19, 45
neomycin 226
neural tube defects (NTDs) 187, 88
neuropsychiatric disorders 142, 246
niacin 155
dietary reference values **155**
safe upper levels 255
nickel 155
interactions 160, 239
safe upper levels 256
nicotinamide 155
action 156
adverse effects 157
safe upper levels 255
nicotinic acid 155, 157
action 156
safe upper levels 255
nitrous oxide 234
non-steroidal anti-inflammatory drugs (NSAIDs) 178
nosebleeds 14
obesity *see* weight management
octacosanol 179
oestrogens 22, 88, 230, 261
older people
fracture prevention 33
immunity 246, 253
muscle strength 64
sleep problems 142
oleic acid 186
oligofructose 230
omega-3 fatty acids 77, 82, 186
omega-6 fatty acids 186
oral contraceptives 261
folic acid interaction 88
pantothenic acid interaction 167
riboflavin interaction 197
vitamin B_{12} interaction 324
vitamin C interaction 239
vitamin E interaction 246
zinc interaction 254
oral hypoglycemics 53, 261
osteoarthritis
boron 22

chondroitin 49
fish oils 79
glucosamine 103
green-lipped mussel 107
methylsulfonylmethane 145
S-adenosyl methionine 201
silicon 210
osteoporosis
calcium 33, 35
fluoride 84
isoflavones 129
melatonin 143
silicon 209
vitamin D 241
vitamin K 249
overweight *see* weight management
oxidative stress 105, 109, 140, 213
see also antioxidants
palmitic acid 186
pangamic acid 163
pantothenic acid 165
dietary reference values **165**
safe upper levels 255
para-amino benzoic acid (PABA) 168
Parkinson's disease 55, 142, 161, 172
penicillamine 62, 126, 231, 254, 262
peptic ulcers 211
periodontal disease 74, 238
peripheral neuropathy 19
peripheral vascular (arterial) disease (PVD) 10, 38, 82, 96
phenobarbital 20, 246
phenothiazines 74, 197, 259
phenytoin 20, 242, 246
phosphatidylcholine (lecithin) 46, 133
phosphatidylserine 172
phosphorus, safe upper levels 255
phylloquinone 248
phytoestrogens 128
phytosterolaemia 175
phytosterols 91, 174
pivampicillin 39
pivmecillanam 39
platelet aggregation 161
PMS *see* premenstrual syndrome
policosanol 161
pollen, bee 13
polyunsaturated fatty acids (PUFAs) 247
see also omega-3 fatty acids; omega-6 fatty acids
potassium 176
dietary reference values **176**
interactions 178, 257, 257
potassium chloride 234
potassium-sparing diuretics 178, 258
pre-eclampsia 8, 33
prebiotics 179
premenstrual syndrome (PMS)
bee pollen 14
dong quai 70
evening primrose oil 73
ginkgo biloba 97
magnesium 137
vitamin B_6 230
pressure ulcers 2
primidone 20, 242
proanthocyanidins 105
probenecid 197
probiotics 181
procyanidins 170
Proprietary Association of Great Britain (PAGB) 264
prostate cancer 33, 8, 242
prostatic hyperplasia, benign (BPH) 13, 186, 187, 253
proton-pump inhibitors 234
psoriasis 1, 61, 79, 82
psyllium 184
pumpkin seeds 186
pycnogenol 170
pyridoxine *see* vitamin B_6
pyrimethamine 88
Quackwatch 266
quercetin 189
4-quinolones 34, 127, 138, 260
Recommended Dietary Allowances (RDAs) viii
Reference Nutrient Intake (RNI) viii

respiratory infections 100, 153, 182
resveratrol 193
retinoids 226
retinol 224
rheumatoid arthritis
 evening primrose oil 74
 fish oil 79
 glucosamine 103
 green-lipped mussel 107
 manganese 140
 selenium 205
riboflavin 195
 dietary reference values **195**
 interactions 22, 197
 safe upper levels 255
 sources 44
rifampicin 261
royal jelly 198
S-adenosyl methionine (SAM) 201, A02.17
Safe Intake, viii, viii
safe upper levels, viii
schizophrenia 79, 190
seasonal affective disorder 96, 142
seasonal allergic rhinitis *see* hay fever
seborrhoeic dermatitis 1
selective serotonin reuptake inhibitors (SSRIs) 118
selenium 203
 action 7, 204
 dietary reference values **203**
 safe upper levels 256
serotonin 117
shark cartilage 207
silicon 209
sinusitis 29
skin conditions 14
sleep disorders 117, 142, 234
soya products 128
sphingomyelin 46
spirulina 211
sports injuries 49, 102
sports performance *see* exercise performance
stannous chloride 219
statins 55, 175, 185, 226
stearic acid 186
stress response 172
stroke 143
sucralfate 226, 242, 246, 250
sulfasalazine 88, 257
sulphonamides 169
sulphur 145
sumatriptan 118
superoxide dismutase (SOD) 213
swelling 29
systemic lupus erythematosus 79
tamoxifen 34
tardive dyskinesia 143
tendonitis 103
tetracyclines 260
 mineral interactions 34, 127, 138, 254
 vitamin C interaction 239
theophylline 231
thiamine 215
 dietary reference values **215**
 safe upper levels 255
thiazide diuretics 34, 138, 178, 242, 257
thioctic acid *see* alpha-lipoic acid
thyroid hormones 122
thyroid medication 123, 262
tin 219
tinnitus 96
tissue growth/repair 44
tocopherols 244
Tolerable Upper Intake Levels (TUL; UL) viii 256
Tonalin 58
tonic 44
toxins, removal 45
tramodol 118
tranquillisers 100
travellers' diarrhoea 181
trazodone 118
tricyclic antidepressants 197
trientine 62, 127
triglycerides 221
trimethoprim 88, 260
tryptophan 157
ubiquinone *see* coenzyme Q10

UL (Tolerable Upper Intake Level) viii 256
ulcerative colitis
aloe vera 2
bromelain 28
fish oil 79
probiotics 182
psyllium 184
United Kingdom
Dietary Reference Values (DRVs) viii
government web sites 263
United States (US)
Dietary Reference Values (DRVs) viii
web sites 263
vaginal yeast infections 181
vanadium 221
interactions 239
safe upper levels 256
venlafaxine 118
venous insufficiency, chronic 29, 103, 105, 170
venous thrombosis, prevention 170
Veris Newsletter, A03.16
vertigo 97
visual acuity 79
vitamin A 224
action 7, 225
deficiency 226
dietary reference values **224**
interactions 226, 239, 247, 250
precursors 40
safe upper levels 255
sources 77
vitamin B_1 *see* thiamine
vitamin B_2 *see* riboflavin
vitamin B_6 (pyrixodine) 228
dietary reference values **228**
drug interactions 230, 258, 259, 260, 261
nutrient interactions 231, 239
safe upper levels 255
vitamin B_{12} 233
deficiency 233
dietary reference values **233**
interactions 234, 239
safe upper levels 255
sources 44
vitamin B_{15} (pangamic acid) 163
vitamin C 236
action 7, 237
bioavailability 8
dietary reference values **236**
drug interactions 238, 261
nutrient interactions 52, 62, 125, 227, 218, 235, 239, 247
safe upper levels 255
vitamin D 240
analogues 242
deficiency 241
dietary reference values **240**
drug interactions 242, 257, 259, 261
nutrient interactions 35, 242
safe upper levels 255
sources 77
vitamin E 244
action 7, 245
bioavailability 8
dietary reference values **244**
drug interactions 246, 258
nutrient interactions 127, 227, 239, 246, 250
safe upper levels 255
sources 77, 186
vitamin K 248
dietary reference values **248**
drug interactions 250, 258, 259
nutrient interactions 227, 247, 250
safe upper levels 256
vitamins
B complex 26, 197, 211, 218, 218
fat-soluble, interactions 175, 257, 259
psyllium interactions 185
safe upper levels 255
warfarin 55, 71, 100, 185
weight management
calcium 33
chitosan 42

conjugated linoleic acid 57
dehydroepiandrosterone 67
green tea extract 109
hydroxycitric acid 115
5-hydroxytryptophan 117
Wernicke–Korsakoff syndrome 218
wine, red 193
World Cancer Research Fund, ix
World Health Organization (WHO) viii, ix
wound healing 1, 10, 44, 238, 253
wound infections 2
yeast, brewers', 26, 259
zeaxanthin 7, 40
zinc 251
action 7, 252
dietary reference values **251**
drug interactions 260, 260, 262
nutrient interactions 35, 62, 88, 127, 247, 254
safe upper levels 256
sources 26, 44
zolpidem 118